About the author

Ger[aldi]ne Miskin is an internationally recognised independent breast-feed[ing] specialist who has over 20 years' experience working with fami[lies] through her private practice in West London, UK.

Wh[ile] studying to become a paediatric nutritionist, Geraldine worked as a [bab]y and maternity nurse before changing her career path. She was ch[osen] out of over 300 applicants to complete a unique 18-month interns[hip] with a leading board-certified lactation consultant, before studyin[g h]uman lactation in depth.

Having s[ee]n first-hand a real need for guidance based on individual circumsta[n]ce, anatomy and lifestyle while working as a maternity nurse, Geraldi[ne] set about learning the science behind breastfeeding, believing that birt[h,] anatomical variations as well as baby's ability to feed, greatly influenc[ed] breastfeeding outcomes.

She devel[op]ed a unique algorithm and methodology called the Miskin Method in 2007. Her practice-based research has deduced two fundam[en]t[a]l points: namely that *babies breastfeed and mums make milk* and that *[milk] is driven by drainage* not demand, which have revolutionised par[ents and] professionals' approach to breastfeeding.

G[eraldine is] the founder and co-owner of Miskin Maternity, an agency [of mat]ernity nurses extensively trained in the Miskin Method and [del]ivers the breastfeeding workshops for the Bump Classes [and Goo]gle.

D0413431

BREASTFEEDING
MADE EASY

Your step-by-step guide to using the

Miskin
Method

GERALDINE MISKIN

Vermilion
LONDON

This is for you, Mom

10 9 8 7 6 5 4 3 2 1

Vermilion, an imprint of Ebury Publishing,
20 Vauxhall Bridge Road,
London SW1V 2SA

Vermilion is part of the Penguin Random House group of companies
whose addresses can be found at global.penguinrandomhouse.com

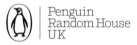

Copyright © Geraldine Miskin 2015
Illustrations Copyright © Geraldine Miskin 2015
Shutterstock Images Copyright © Shutterstock, Inc. 2015

Geraldine Miskin has asserted her right to be identified
as the author of this Work in accordance with the Copyright, Designs
and Patents Act 1988

All rights reserved. No part of this publication may be reproduced,
stored in a retrieval system, or transmitted in any form or by any means,
including digital, electronic, mechanical, photocopying, recording or otherwise,
without the prior permission of the copyright owner.

First published by Vermilion in 2015

www.eburypublishing.co.uk

A CIP catalogue record for this book is available from the British Library

ISBN 9781785040122

Printed and bound in China by C&C Offset Printing Co., Ltd

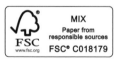

Penguin Random House is committed to a sustainable
future for our business, our readers and our planet.
This book is made from Forest Stewardship
Council® certified paper.

The information in this book has been compiled by way of general guidance in relation to the
specific subjects addressed, but is not a substitute and not to be relied on for medical, healthcare,
pharmaceutical or other professional advice on specific circumstances and in specific locations. So far
as the author is aware the information given is correct and up to date as at January 2015. Practice,
laws and regulations all change, and the reader should obtain up to date professional advice on any
such issues. The author and publishers disclaim, as far as the law allows, any liability arising directly or
indirectly from the use, or misuse, of the information contained in this book.

FOREWORD

The benefits of breastfeeding are well documented and extend to both new mother and her baby, lasting for years beyond the breastfeeding period and even into adulthood. Breastfeeding plays an incredibly important part in determining and contributing to a young baby's health. It reinforces and promotes bonding by frequent contact between mum and baby and provides protection against infections, as well as individually tailored nutrition.

Breastfeeding has played a prominent role in many communities around the world throughout history and appears to come more easily if the new mother is well supported by her extended family. The family provides structure, wisdom and role models; enabling her to gain the confidence and skills she needs to breastfeed.

In today's society, many new mums don't have this close-knit network around them, often living far from their extended families. As a result, they have fewer examples of successful breastfeeding, less support and greater pressure to get breastfeeding right on their own.

In this book, Geraldine Miskin shares her expert experience, skills and unique Miskin Method, combining the science and art of breastfeeding and putting both into practice. Her advice, understanding, top tips and clear illustrations will help mums and babies to calmly overcome any difficulties and go on to enjoy and benefit from successful breastfeeding.

Dr Ian Hay
Consultant Paediatrician
MMed, FCP(SA), FRCPCH

TABLE OF CONTENTS

THE MISKIN METHOD IN A NUTSHELL

When there are so many breastfeeding books on the shelf already, why do you need to read this one?

Firstly, I see you as an individual and, while it is essential that your new baby gets everything that he needs, I believe it is paramount that your needs are also considered and met. My method, the Miskin Method, is a mum-and-baby-focused approach. It's gentle enough to use from birth and pragmatic to ensure that you get great results. This is how and why I'm different.

Secondly, in these pages you will learn how everything works and fits together – as well as what you can do if it doesn't. Background information is key to guiding you towards choices and solutions that will make your breastfeeding experience wonderful, effective and rewarding.

Thirdly, the Miskin Method is a fresh, flexible and practical approach that is based on five key elements that I will briefly outline here. I'm not trying to turn you into a breastfeeding specialist, but I want to give you an insight into how five individual elements can transform your breastfeeding experience.

THE FIVE KEY ELEMENTS OF THE MISKIN METHOD

I see the five key elements of my method as similar to five baking ingredients that we all have at home – namely milk, butter, eggs, flour and sugar.

You can combine these ingredients in different ways to make delicious cakes, biscuits and puddings, then, once you have got the basics right, you can add cocoa, vanilla extract, nuts, coconut flakes or anything else you can think of to make the recipe 'yours'. Breastfeeding is just the same, and these are the five ingredients you need to consider when creating your perfect breastfeeding 'recipe'. As with baking, once you've mastered the breastfeeding basics you can adapt them to suit you and your baby as he develops and grows.

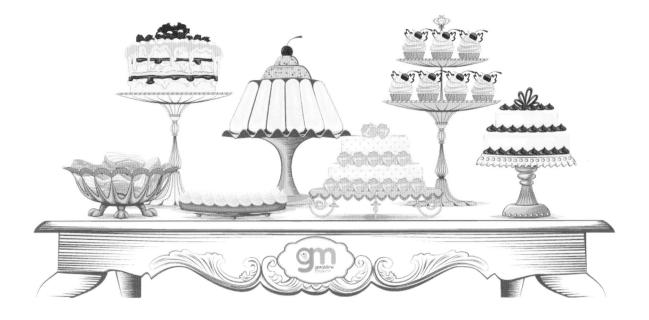

1 You

It all starts with you, so decide what you'd like to achieve and find out how to do it before your baby arrives. If by nature you like routine, follow a routine. If you don't like structure, don't bother with routines. Either way is fine.

Your breast shape and size will influence all of your decisions – such as how often to feed and whether to offer one or both sides at each feed (see page 79). Your breast and nipple will indicate how you should position baby at your breast and latch him in order to ensure that breastfeeding is comfortable for you both (see page 38). And, lastly, these physical components will also determine how easy expressing milk will be (see page 98).

2 Baby

The size of baby's mouth and the shape of his palate affect how much breast tissue he can scoop up when he latches (see page 52). This in turn determines how well you and baby fit together and how easily he can access your milk.

3 Baby's age and size

Your baby's age influences his ability to breastfeed and how much energy he has to do it. There will also be milestones as his gets older – such as growth spurts – when you should expect his feeding patterns to change (see page 82). Your baby's size typically indicates his tummy capacity, however some tiny babies drink much more than babies double their size, so always follow your baby's lead and monitor his weight gain (see page 77).

4 Your medical history

Your medical history will indicate whether or not there are concerns about milk production. If you don't have an underlying medical condition that reduces supply, you will have enough milk for your baby (see page 21).

5 Labour and birth

As your baby goes through labour and birth, he gets pushed, squeezed and turned until he is born. Understandably he may feel stiff or tight by the end of it. Tightness affects how comfortable baby is in a certain position, how wide he opens his mouth and how easily he is able to transfer your breast milk. This tightness is only temporary, but it can make your early feeds tricky (see page 139).

11

These five essential breastfeeding ingredients vary quite a bit between mums and babies – you only have to look at your friends to see how different they and their babies are to you and your baby.

Breastfeeding can and will work for you when you consider and embrace your uniqueness. Current breastfeeding rates prove that the stale, one-size-fits-all, bog-standard advice doesn't work. It's time to get personal – and this book will give you the skills to do just that.

10 GOLDEN BREASTFEEDING RULES

These are my top 10 practical tips that will transform your breastfeeding experience and give you confidence to know that everything is going well right from the start.

1   Aim for an off-centre latch (*Fig. 1*)
Rather than aiming for a bulls-eye latch with your nipple in the centre, aim for an off-centre latch that looks like this. Your nipple will be out of the way and baby will get your milk really easily (see page 52).

2   Bring baby to the breast quickly when latching
The quicker your nipple gets to the back of baby's mouth, the more comfortable the latch will be. You only have a very small window of opportunity to get your breast to where it needs to be before baby starts to close his mouth (see page 27).

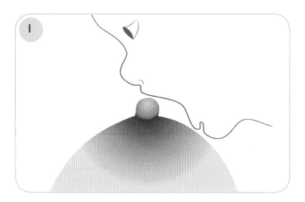

3   Watch for swallows rather than watching the clock
When feeding, focus on how often your baby swallows, rather than how long he feeds for. It is much better for your baby to swallow frequently and feed for 10 minutes than suck for ages before swallowing and so stretch out the feed for 60 minutes. (See page 29 for tips on monitoring swallows.)

4   Keep feeds effective
It's lovely to have baby at your breast, but if he constantly snoozes, you'll be there all day.
   Breast compression delivers milk into your baby's mouth, keeping him awake and ensuring he feeds effectively. It is a much better technique to use to keep him feeding efficiently than blowing on his face or tickling his feet. (See page 21 for advice on how to do it.)

5   Wake to feed for better nights
Your baby will sleep well at night if he gets the bulk of his milk during the day. If your baby doesn't wake on his own for daytime feeds and prefers to feed more at night, you can wake him and feed him during the daytime to encourage him to sleep better at night. (See page 113.)

6 **Feed according to your anatomy**

Your breast size doesn't determine how much milk you produce in 24 hours but it does influence how much milk you produce in one go. To ensure your baby gets enough milk over the course of the day you need to feed in line with your cup size to maintain a healthy supply (see page 79).

7 **Monitor poo and weight gain to know what's going in**

In the first week, before you are able to weigh him regularly, you can track the changes to baby's poo to see that he is getting enough colostrum. This will give you confidence that he is getting what he needs, even if you feel as if you don't have much to offer him. (See page 70.)

After the first week, you will know that your baby is getting enough milk if he gains the expected amount of weight. Further more, the extent of his weight gain will tell you whether he is feeding enough, too much or not enough. (See page 78 for weight gain information.)

8 **Feed regularly to establish a pattern**

When you feed at regular intervals, your body knows what to expect and milk production will be really straightforward. As much as possible, find a feeding pattern or rhythm that works for you and baby and stick to it.

9 **Make more milk**

Any milk that you drain from the breast is automatically replaced. To make more milk, feed more often or express if baby is not feeding well. Any breast that makes some milk can make more milk. (For the skinny on low supply, see page 159.)

10 **Give up breastfeeding on a 'good day'**

When you give up on a 'good day' you know that you have done your best and exhausted all your options. Don't give up breastfeeding when you are at your lowest ebb because then you'll wonder whether you gave up too soon and in the heat of the moment. Give breastfeeding your best shot and know when to call it a day without feeling any guilt. (See page 125 for how to wean baby off the breast.)

13

HOW TO USE THIS BOOK

Whether this is your first, second or third baby, this book will help you prepare for breastfeeding. It will be an invaluable reference tool from birth and as your baby grows because it was written with you in mind.

You are looking for a book about breastfeeding because it is important to you; you want to do your very best for your baby and you want to make sure that you know how to breastfeed from the start. You know that many babies breastfeed well and without any problem but you want to be prepared and confident about your role as a mother, so that you can enjoy feeding and caring for your baby.

You have probably heard from friends – or learnt from previous experience – that breastfeeding doesn't always come naturally, and when it goes wrong, it's difficult to find solutions that work when you are sifting through tons of conflicting advice.

The truth is that many mums struggle with breastfeeding because they don't understand that 80 per cent of breastfeeding success is down to what your baby does or doesn't do at the breast.

There is so much conflicting advice about breastfeeding because until now there has not been an algorithm available that takes your uniqueness into account; one that will ensure that you are given information relevant to you and your baby instead of a one-size-fits-all version.

So I have written this book to help you give breastfeeding your best shot. It's packed with practical knowledge that I've distilled from over two decades of helping thousands of mums feed their babies. There are tons of full-colour diagrams to help you see solutions quickly and easily, and alternative options to try when one doesn't work for you and your baby.

Relevant chapters are grouped together so that you can find all the information you need in one area easily within a few pages, with the 'nuts and bolts' chapters placed right at the start so they can be found in a hurry.

I've dedicated a large chunk of the book to troubleshooting chapters, not because I expect you to have problems but because I know that when it isn't easy, you need as much insight and practical help as possible to get breastfeeding right.

There are also useful products and services lists for you to look at before your baby arrives. You don't need much if breastfeeding is going well but it's helpful to know what's available, as well as how and when to use products if breastfeeding isn't straightforward and you need a little help.

If you are lucky enough to be reading this book before baby arrives (and do try to – it's good to be prepared), familiarise yourself with the first six chapters as a priority. Then take this book into hospital with you when the big day comes, so that you can create good habits right from the start. Once baby arrives, you can dip in and out of these chapters until you feel these steps are second nature.

I've done my very best to make this book as practical as possible and not preachy, and I hope it will soon become your very breast friend.

PART 1:
GETTING STARTED

CHAPTER 1

BREAST MILK AND ANATOMY
DESIGNED TO SATISFY

You have cared for and nurtured your baby for months while he was developing in your womb. Now, as your baby comes into the outside world, your body is perfectly capable and ready to continue its role in providing all the nutrients he needs.

The close contact with you that breastfeeding brings makes him feel secure in unfamiliar surroundings, and because he gets this sense of security with each feed, this strong and safe bond is reinforced repeatedly throughout the day, every day.

Your breast milk is a unique source of food; it is packed with anti-infective and growth-promoting components, enzymes to aid digestion in an immature gut, fatty acids that are important for brain development and a vast array of nutritive properties. There is nothing like it; your milk is an incredible living fluid which is not only species- and family-specific (did you know that your milk matches 50 per cent of your baby's genetic make-up?) but also environment-specific, and its make-up changes frequently throughout the day.

Your breastfeeding relationship is designed to keep you and your baby together, so take the pressure off yourself to get baby sleeping through the night as soon as possible and try to enjoy being a mum and just getting to know him.

A good breastfeeding experience is largely based on the confidence you have in your body's ability to provide what your baby needs.

How it all works

Your body is primed to produce milk as soon and as often as your baby needs it – before he even asks for it. In fact, you are so in tune with your baby that he can trigger a milk 'let-down' by crying, rooting, foraging for the nipple and suckling.

Without you doing anything special, your body releases milk in response to your baby's needs and in readiness for a feed. During the feed, you continue to produce and release milk until your baby is full, satisfied and looks blissed out and drunk on your milk.

TIP

If you have too much milk your baby will nipple-feed and avoid your areola to regulate the flow.

↪ Changes to breast size and shape during pregnancy

During pregnancy, your glandular tissue or milk-producing tissue develops in preparation for breastfeeding. This often alters your breast size or shape and is usually the first indicator that you are pregnant.

Ordinarily it is fat that gives your breast shape and contributes to its size, and as the fat in your breast is replaced by glandular tissue, you'll feel that your breasts are heavier but not much bigger. It is only when the glandular tissue develops and the fatty tissue stays put that you are most likely to notice an increase in your breast size.

↪ Change in breast firmness

More often than not, the fat in your breast is replaced by milk-producing tissue that develops during pregnancy, irrespective of whether or not you choose to breastfeed. Breastfeeding per se isn't responsible for changes in the shape of your breasts; because fat gives your breast shape, after pregnancy or when you stop feeding your breasts may feel softer and look flatter as the fat as been replaced by milk-producing breast tissue.

17

What your breast looks like inside

Your breast is essentially made up of four parts: alveoli or milk sacs, milk ducts, fat and connective ligaments. Imagine the inside of the breast as a bit like a bush; the nipple is the stump of the bush, the milk ducts are the branches, and the clusters of alveoli are the leaves.

↝ The milk duct system
Your milk ducts carry milk from the alveoli to the nipple. Small ducts connected to your milk sacs feed into larger ducts that deliver milk to your baby via your nipple. They are naturally collapsed and only dilate or open to allow milk flow.

↝ Nipple pores
Pores or tiny openings found on the tip of your nipple deliver your milk into baby's mouth. On average, you will have between 4 and 12 pores on each breast. The pores are mostly found on the nipple tip but sometimes they can also be found on the areola.

↝ Milk-producing sacs (alveoli)
You won't be able to feel individual milk sacs in your breasts because they are tiny and group together to form pea-size clusters. You can often feel these clusters when your breast is full or just before a feed.

Your alveoli are lined with milk-producing cells called lactocytes. Milk is produced in these special cells and then stored inside your milk sacs in readiness for a feed.

The majority of your milk-producing tissue is found within a 3cm radius from the base of the nipple.

18

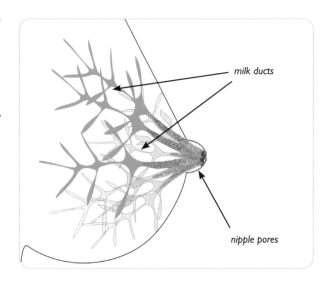

milk ducts

nipple pores

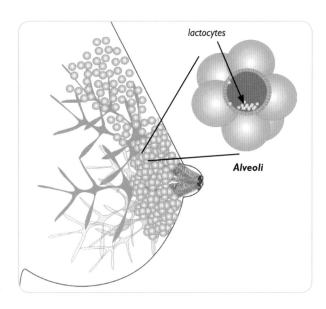

lactocytes

Alveoli

How milk is made

To make milk you need two hormones: prolactin and oxytocin. While these two hormones work together to make and deliver milk, each have their own individual roles. Prolactin is responsible for milk production and oxytocin ensures that your alveoli contract and release your milk.

In order to work, each hormone needs receptor cells located where the hormone is used. Prolactin receptor cells are found next to milk-producing cells (lactocytes) and oxytocin receptor cells are found next to the contractile unit of your milk sacs, or alveoli.

The receptor cells are dormant but are activated by feeds in the early days. The more baby feeds, the more receptor cells become active and the more effective your hormones are.

Each alveolus or milk sac has a band of muscles called a contractile unit. These muscles are in a relaxed state while your milk sacs fill up. (*Fig. 1*)

When baby suckles, your body releases oxytocin, which causes the muscles around your milk sacs to contract and squeeze out the milk. This release of milk is what we call a let-down. Once your milk sacs are empty, they pop open and start refilling again, in readiness for the next let-down. (*Fig. 2*)

You will have between two and five let-downs in both breasts simultaneously during a feed, which feels like a tingling sensation. Sometimes the tingling is so subtle that you don't even notice that you have had a let-down until you see the second side leaking.

19

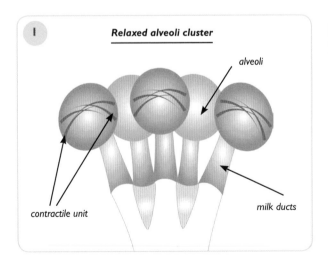

1 *Relaxed alveoli cluster*

alveoli

contractile unit

milk ducts

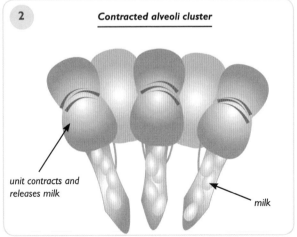

2 *Contracted alveoli cluster*

unit contracts and releases milk

milk

↪ Milk stream

The more glandular tissue you have, the more milk you will release in one go. This continuous spray is what I refer to as a milk stream. The longer your milk stream continues, the longer your baby has to swallow without breathing before he gets a natural break. You may be told that your baby is 'hungry' or 'greedy' if he gulps your milk down, but milk flow has more to do with the force of your let-down than how 'greedy' your baby is.

↪ How foremilk and hind milk are made

This sounds complicated, but it is actually very simple. When your body makes milk it starts by producing a calorie-rich milk and then water is drawn into the alveoli to dilute the concentrate and increase the volume of milk produced.

Your milk is watery at the start of the feed because your alveoli have had plenty of time to draw water in between the end of the last feed and the start of the next. This milk is called foremilk because it is the milk your baby gets at the start of the feed.

As your alveoli empty and refill during the feed, your milk becomes creamier as there is less time available to draw water in between let-downs. This is called the hind milk because it is the milk your baby gets at the end of the feed.

TIP

During growth spurts your baby feeds frequently in order to access the calorie-rich milk before it dilutes so that he can facilitate his exaggerated period of growth. How clever is that?

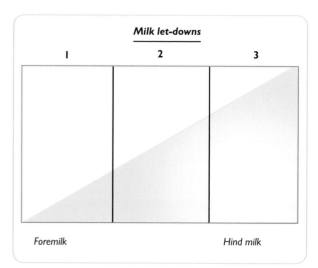

The influences on supply and flow

⇥ How your body reduces milk supply

Your body needs to regulate the milk you supply so that your baby gets a good balance of fore and hind milk at each feed. Again, your body has a very clever way of doing this and it is all down to a protein in your milk called FIL – feedback inhibiter of lactation.

As your milk is made, molecules of FIL enter your alveoli. The amount of FIL in your milk sacs is proportionate to the amount of milk produced, so when your milk sacs are empty, there is little or no FIL present, but as your alveoli fill up, the number of FIL molecules increases too.

High levels of FIL in your milk relay a message to your brain to slow down or stop milk production completely. This way, your body is able to provide what your baby needs while ensuring that you don't become overfull. So, provided you feed frequently and before your breast becomes overly full, you'll always have enough milk for him.

⇥ How to increase your milk flow artificially

There are times when you need to increase your milk flow to make breastfeeding more effective or to encourage your baby to stay awake and keep feeding, especially in the early days. The easiest and most effective way to do this is to compress your breast with a flat hand so that you are literally manually squeezing milk out of your alveoli to create a let-down. I call this breast compression – I will refer to it a lot throughout this book because it is pure gold!

Place a flat hand on your breast and push inwards towards your ribcage. (*Fig. 1*) Ensure that your hand is not too close to your nipple or you will pull it out of baby's mouth. Push in and hold for 20 seconds – or until he starts swallowing – then stop. Work your way around the breast to drain it completely.

This is one of my top tips because it works within seconds and is very effective. You can forget about blowing on or tickling your baby to keep him awake; just compress your breast and he will get milk delivered into his mouth and will keep feeding.

Only compress if your baby needs help getting your milk. Don't compress if he is already swallowing as this can lead to your flow overwhelming him and result in unnecessary trapped wind.

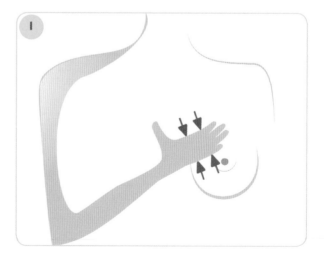

Milk tailored to your baby's needs

Your milk spontaneously goes through many changes from baby's birth all the way through to weaning, without any input from you.

↪ First milk

In preparation for breastfeeding, you produce colostrum from week 12 of pregnancy, beginning with tiny amounts. The hormone progesterone restricts overall production, but you may notice a sticky residue on your bra from week 16 if you produce a lot of colostrum and leak. Once your baby is born, colostrum is produced in abundance, which is perfectly tailored to his needs.

It's designed with baby in mind

Colostrum is high in protein, antioxidants, growth promoters, immune-boosting properties, enzymes, white blood cells, laxative properties, vitamins A and E and also carotenoids, which give it its yellow colour. Colostrum is packed with goodness and not much fluid; these small portions are perfect for your baby's tiny tummy (which is the size of a Malteser when he is born) and his immature kidneys because they aren't able to tolerate large volumes yet.

It supports baby's immature digestive system

Colostrum protects your baby from infections and developing sensitivities by painting a protective lining on the walls of your baby's gut, making it less permeable. This protective lining restricts pathogens being absorbed into your baby's body.

It reduces jaundice symptoms

When your baby is born, he breaks down excess red blood cells that he no longer needs. The waste product of this process is bilirubin and the quickest way to get rid of it is for baby to poo like a champ. Your colostrum is an effective laxative, so the more he gets, the more he poos and the quicker he becomes jaundice-free.

How your milk changes

Your milk changes in line with your baby's developmental milestones in order to meet and satisfy his growing needs.

↠ **Colostrum (days 0, 1 and 2) *(Fig. 1)***

Once your placenta is delivered, the progesterone responsible for suppressing milk production during pregnancy drops. Immediately after birth your baby will receive the colostrum that is ready and waiting in your breasts.

Your thick colostrum flows slowly, which gives him a chance to practise how to suck, swallow and breathe – something he hasn't had to do before now. Your breasts won't feel very different yet because the volume of colostrum produced is tiny. Your colostrum will quickly begin to increase and dilute in order to satisfy your baby's growing appetite.

If you have a tough labour or an eventful delivery, your colostrum may be slow to dilute and increase. This is normal and is your body's way of recovering while feeding baby. If your baby seems a bit hungry, just offer the breast more frequently and your supply will soon increase to meet his needs. (See page 21.)

↠ **Transitional milk (days 3 to 14) *(Fig. 2)***

By day 3 or 4, your colostrum has become runny and yellow in colour. This is what I call transitional milk – the milk that is produced in between colostrum and mature milk. You won't notice this change unless you leak or baby brings up his feed.

The components are primarily the same as colostrum, so it's important that baby continues to get as much opportunity to feed as possible. The more he gets, the more he will poo and the quicker he will get rid of any lingering jaundice while also enjoying all the health benefits of your milk.

With the influx of this transitional milk, your breasts may feel full, hot and achy. This fullness is often referred to as engorgement, or your milk 'coming in' (see page 131).

Even though your milk is runny, it is not mature milk yet so you don't have to worry about baby 'getting to the hind milk' at each feed. Your transitional milk will continue to dilute until it is mature milk – between days 10 and 14.

23

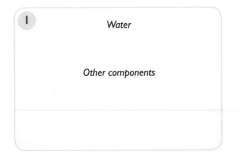

1

Water

Other components

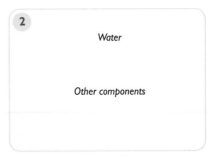

2

Water

Other components

↬ Mature milk (day 14) (*Fig. 3*)

Towards the end of the second week, your transitional milk has diluted to become mature milk. Your milk is now white instead of yellow and appears more watery at the start of the feed (the foremilk) and creamier at the end of it (the hind milk).

Your milk continues to provide the nutrients, immune-boosting properties, fatty acids for brain development and pretty much anything else your baby needs.

You'll know that he is getting enough hind milk if his poos become and remain yellow after day 10.

PEAK AND DIP OF MILK SUPPLY

Your milk peaks and dips at different times of the day. It is at its greatest quantity between 1am and 4am and lowest between 1pm and 4pm. Morning feeds are usually quicker as there is more milk available, while afternoon feeds are close together as your baby cluster feeds to get enough milk before night-time.

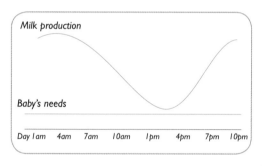

Milk production

Baby's needs

Day 1am 4am 7am 10am 1pm 4pm 7pm 10pm

3

Water

Other components

How diet, alcohol and exercise affect breastfeeding

➝ Diet

What you eat is important to ensure that you stay healthy while you are taking care of all your baby's needs. Your milk will be perfect regardless of whether you eat well or not, but by eating healthily you will be better able to cope with all of the intense demands of being a mum.

Proper meals are important, but make sure you eat small snacks throughout the day, too, to balance your blood sugar levels, keep cravings at bay and give you energy. Choose foods that convert to energy slowly, such as oats, rather than relying on sugar hits to give you a lift.

Certain foods, such as coconut oil, mackerel, salmon, dark green leafy vegetables, apricots, almonds and lentils, will boost the quality of your milk. You need an additional 700 calories a day to produce enough milk to feed baby, so while you may want to get back into your pre-pregnancy wardrobe as soon as possible, don't cut back on calories too quickly. (See the Contented Calf recipe book for easy, tasty lactogenic recipes that are calorific and healthy to get you started, page 186.)

➝ Water

You need to ensure that you drink enough water to remain hydrated as well as maintaining an abundant supply. Aim to have at least one glass of water with each feed.

➝ Alcohol

One small glass of wine with dinner once or twice a week is not necessarily going to affect breastfeeding. Have a small glass of wine and monitor how well your baby feeds afterwards and whether it causes him discomfort. Provided he is unaffected – and you don't drink every night or go overboard when you do – you can enjoy a glass without feeling guilty.

➝ Exercise

You can get back into a regular exercise routine after week 6, but when you do, take it easy. Don't do any more than 45 minutes of moderate exercise twice a week to start with. You can gradually build this up to five times a week but you don't want to over-exert yourself as this will suppress your supply – especially at 12 weeks when your supply dips naturally. (See page 177.)

From the moment your baby is born, you are able to give him what he requires in perfectly sized portions to meet his growing needs. As these needs change, your supply will too. Your baby also does his bit and the next chapter will explain exactly what he expects to happen as he grows and develops.

CHAPTER 2

HOW YOUR BABY BREASTFEEDS
WHAT YOUR BABY WANTS YOU TO KNOW

While your body readies itself for birth and milk production, your baby is practising the skills he will need outside the womb by learning to swallow amniotic fluid and suckling on his thumb. His input is very important to breastfeeding, as success is largely based on how well he breastfeeds.

Your baby's reflexes and instincts help him find and latch on to the breast when left to his own devices. Some of these may seem to make breastfeeding harder for you, but when you understand why he flaps his arms around or squeals in frustration you can improvise and find ways to accommodate his innate reflexes and keep feeding times calm.

What your baby expects to happen when he feeds

Your baby's head is heavy and his neck muscles weak when he is first born. In order for him to lift his head to search or root for your nipple, he needs to steady himself. When you lie back and put him tummy to tummy with you, his body has maximum contact with your body, which provides the best source of stability.

In this position your baby is able to mobilise himself so that he can find and latch on to your breast. He uses his legs to propel himself forwards and once he locates a nipple, he uses his hands to tweak it so that it becomes erect, as well as shape your breast so that it is easier for him to latch.

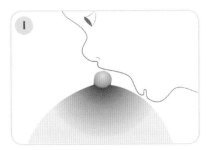

→ Your baby needs to be in an off-centre position so that he gets more areola close to his lower lip into his mouth. (*Fig. 1*)

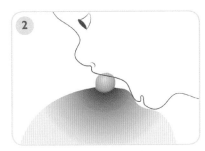

→ As he latches, his chin makes first contact with your breast. His tongue will come down and forward to pad his lower gum and create space in his mouth for your breast. The pressure of his chin coming into the breast tilts your nipple downwards so that it just skims under his top lip. (*Fig. 2*)

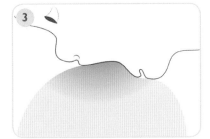

→ He gets a good mouthful of breast and your nipple ends up at the back of his mouth where it won't get damaged. (*Fig. 3*)

27

How he gets your milk

When your baby suckles, his tongue moves in a wave-like, lapping motion, compressing your breast against the roof of his mouth.

He creates suction to keep your breast in place by doing a sequence of quick sucks. When your milk comes down, his sucking pattern changes from being constantly quick to more of a suck, suck, swallow pattern.

To draw milk into his mouth, he drops his tongue and lower jaw, which creates a stronger vacuum and larger oral space. Your milk sprays into his mouth and his tongue guides it to the back of his mouth where he will swallow it.

He maintains an airtight latch and begins suckling again to draw more milk from the breast.

Watch your baby to see if he is swallowing regularly (*see below*). If you look down at baby, watch his double chin and you will notice that when he sucks his jaw moves up and down really quickly.

When he swallows, his jaw drops a fraction lower and pauses for a split second before he starts sucking again.

You can also listen for swallows. You may hear gulping if your flow is fast or you may just hear a subtle exhalation from his nose with each swallow. If you aren't sure what I mean, have a sip of water and listen for the exhalation from your nose just after you swallow.

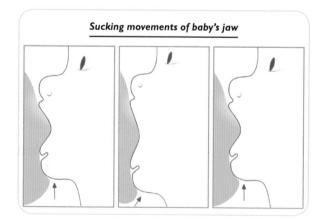

Sucking movements of baby's jaw

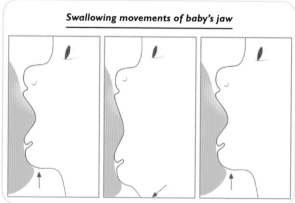

Swallowing movements of baby's jaw

Swallows tell you he's getting milk

The best way to know if your baby is getting any milk is to look for swallows. The more frequently he swallows, the quicker his feed will be over. The more he sucks before he swallows, the harder he is working and the longer his feeds will take.

The better able he is to transfer milk, the better your supply will be and the less energy he will use during the feed. Ideally you want to see that he does one to two sucks per swallow at the start of the feed. This tells you that your supply is great and he can get the milk easily.

If he does 10 sucks per swallow, you know that your supply is low or that he is not transferring well. (See page 158 for tips on low supply, or page 21 to learn about breast compression.)

TIP

If you want some visual guidance to make sure you can tell the difference between sucks and swallows, google 'Dr Jack Newman breastfeeding videos' and you'll find lots of footage showing babies swallowing during their feed.

Over time you will instinctively know whether your baby has had a good or bad feed. Until you have a better idea of what is normal for him, monitor his swallows. It's normal for your supply to fluctuate during the day. This will change the length and effectiveness of feeds, but as long as your baby gets what he needs in a 24-hour period, there is no need to worry about these minor differences.

Your breast size influences breastfeeds in many ways too and I will explain what to expect based on your breast shape and size in the next chapter.

CHAPTER 3

HOW BREAST SIZE AND SHAPE INFLUENCE BREASTFEEDING
YOUR FOUNDATION BLOCKS

By the time your baby is born, all the foundations for successful breastfeeding are in place. However your milk supply is largely based on how much your baby drains from the breast. The more frequently and effectively he drains your breast, the more you will produce. While your breast size doesn't determine how much milk you will produce in a day, it does indicate how much storage capacity you have, how quickly you will fill up and therefore how often you will need to feed before FIL steps in to decrease your production. (See page 21.)

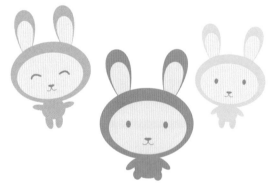

Different-sized breasts

↝ Small breasts (AA–D)

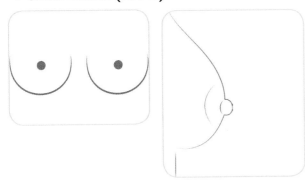

Small breasts typically have less glandular tissue than larger breasts, so naturally they will produce smaller amounts of milk at a time. You will still produce enough milk for your baby, but you may need to feed often to ensure that he meets his daily calorie quota.

Your breasts may feel tight when your milk first comes in, as your breast size doesn't allow for a great deal of flexibility to cope with an influx of milk. As your storage capacity is restricted, you may not be able to go for hours between feeds without experiencing discomfort, especially at night when your supply is at its highest. If you don't feed often and your breasts are full for long periods your supply will drop due to FIL increasing in your milk (see page 21). Feed as soon as your breasts have refilled to prompt more production.

Common challenges

Fast flow – As there just isn't much space in your breasts, you are likely to have a fast, forceful spray. The build-up of pressure in the breast needs a quick release, and this often leads to a flustered feed and a slightly overwhelmed baby.

Shallow latch – When your baby is faced with a fast flow, the natural thing for him to do is to pull back, away from the breast and on to the nipple. While this may be better for baby, a shallow latch can cause you nipple soreness (see page 142).

Windy baby – A fast, forceful spray often leads to baby swallowing a lot of wind during the feed which accumulates during the day and results in colicky behaviour in the evening. Excessive wind intake can also lead to him feeling full before he really is, preventing him from draining your breast fully. You'll find that he asks for milk soon after the last feed, which often seems to make matters worse. (See page 58 for essential winding tips.)

Poor breast drainage – This is a by-product of baby taking in a lot of wind and feeling full before he really is (see page 154 and also page 181 for information on taking lecithin to help this).

Low milk supply – Provided you feed frequently during the day and wind effectively at each feed, you are no more likely to suffer low supply than anyone else.

➡ Medium-sized breasts (DD–G)

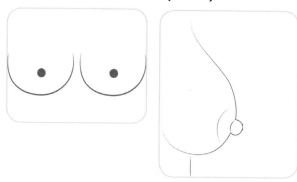

You are in a pretty 'stable' zone with regards to glandular tissue and milk production. As such, you'll have a greater degree of flexibility to cope with an influx of milk and may even feel comfortable when your baby sleeps for longer stretches at night.

Your breasts aren't as sensitive to small changes in breast drainage or ad hoc feeding patterns as small breasts are, but it is worth getting into a good feeding rhythm anyway.

Common challenges

Breast growth – If you have gone from an A cup to an EE during pregnancy, you may feel like you don't recognise the two foreign objects attached to your chest. This is more of a personal comfort challenge than a breastfeeding challenge but it is worth mentioning.

It is important to purchase and wear a bra that is well-fitting and supports your newly larger breasts. When your breasts are heavy and full of milk, extra support prevents ligaments in the breast stretching and your breast tissue sagging. It always helps if you get a style you like and feel good in, too.

Too much milk – A considerable increase in breast size usually indicates that your glandular tissue has increased and that you will produce a lot of milk. Feed regularly to avoid unnecessary engorgement and a forceful let-down.

Prolonged milk stream – Your baby may struggle with your milk stream, especially if he is little. As he gets bigger, feeding will get easier and he will learn to cope with your flow. Until then, manage your flow by using some of the tips on page 48.

32

TIP

Don't worry if your breasts feel empty before feeds. This is normal when you have enough storage capacity for milk.

↝ Large breasts (GG+)

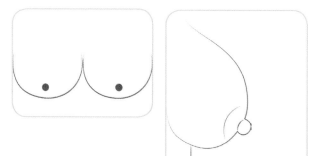

If you have large breasts they may feel like moving targets, which makes latching and keeping them in baby's mouth a bit of a challenge. However, you will see the full benefit of having larger breasts when your baby's stomach capacity increases sufficiently to hold enough milk to enable him to sleep for hours at night.

Common challenges

Comfort – Get a good bra and ensure that you like the style and feel comfortable. You need good support or your breasts and back will take the strain and start to ache.

Forceful let-down – As you have a lot of glandular tissue, your baby will be hit with a wall of milk seconds after latching. Calm your flow by feeding in specific positions (see page 47).

Prolonged milk stream – Manage your milk stream and take him off the breast to create short breaks to enable him to catch his breath. If you have a 'jet' stream and he struggles to breathe, you'll need to change your feeding position too (see page 47).

Great pretenders – Some large breasts give the impression of having a lot of glandular tissue when in fact the breast is primarily made up of fat. Just be aware that not all large breasts automatically indicate excess milk production or storage capacity. Always monitor baby's nappies and weight gain to be sure that he is getting enough milk. If his weight gain is slow, follow the breastfeeding rules for small-breasted mums.

33

> TIP
>
> You'll soon be the envy of your friends when your baby sleeps for longer stretches and gains weight by the bucketload.

Different-shaped breasts

➥ **Uneven breasts**

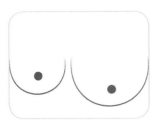

It's normal for one breast to be slightly bigger than the other, but when one breast is three sizes smaller than the other, you will find that supply is very uneven and there is a notable difference in storage capacity.

Feed from both sides at each feed rather than trying to feed from one side each time. Start on the smaller side in the morning when your supply is highest and on the bigger side at feeds when your supply is lower.

Any breast that makes milk can make more milk, so persevere with breastfeeding on your small side and supply will increase.

TIP

Use your high-production periods to counterbalance your low ones. See page 98 for advice on how to express milk and accumulate it for a bottle feed.

Common challenges

Uneven production – Uneven production levels make it tricky to get into a 'standard' breastfeeding pattern, so to start with just focus on getting your supply established (see page 158). It is important to ensure that your smaller breast is never full for too long or your supply will drop.

Low milk supply – You may be worried about how much you'll be able to produce if one breast is very small. The upside is that you have one small and one medium-to-large breast and this will make it easier than breastfeeding with two small breasts. Don't be put off and give breastfeeding a go.

Feeling lopsided – As your glandular tissue builds up to full production mode, you may notice the difference in size between your two breasts. This is easily resolved by using bra inserts to even out the smaller side.

Expressing – You may find it more challenging on one side than the other due to different degrees of storage capacity. Give it a go anyway and have a look at expressing tips for small-breasted mums so that you can make the most of your available glandular tissue (see page 103).

➦ Tubular breasts

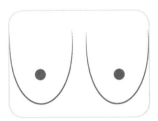

Tubular breasts, which are elongated and tubular in shape rather than round, need to be monitored carefully as they often coincide with low-milk-supply issues. In this situation, more care needs to be taken to ensure that your baby gets what he needs from the breast.

The easiest way to do this is to monitor his poos, pees and weight gain. This is the only way to know for sure that your baby is getting enough milk, regardless of your bra size or shape.

Common challenges

Absence of breast growth during pregnancy – As this shape poses a concern, you want to see growth during pregnancy. An absence of growth or change in shape could indicate that you are more vulnerable to low-supply issues than other mums, so monitor baby's weight gain closely.

Low milk supply – Follow the rules for small-breasted mums until your supply is established. (Also see page 158 for tips on how to boost your supply.)

Expressing – As with small-breasted mums, you may find expressing a bit of a chore because you won't have excess milk available to express after baby has had his fill. (See expressing tips for small-breasted mums, page 103.)

Supplements – If your supply is low, you'll need to give baby formula start-up or top ups to make breastfeeding as efficient as possible. (See page 107.)

Surgery – If you have had corrective surgery, feed, feed, feed to boost and maintain your supply. It will feel relentless to start with but it will be really worth it in the end.

TIP

Any breast milk your baby gets will boost his health. Add in a bottle of formula if you have to, knowing that your baby is still getting the very best you can offer.

Breast surgery

↪ Breast implants

If you have had breast implants, it's good to know that this surgery doesn't usually interfere with the development of your glandular tissue, but the implants themselves will restrict your storage capacity quite a bit. You will be able to feed baby really well but you need to follow the rules for small-breasted mums. If you have had significant breast growth during pregnancy, though, follow the rules for medium-breasted mums.

Common challenges

Engorgement – As the storage capacity in your breast is reduced by the implant, you could feel quite sore when your milk comes in. This sensation should settle down within a few days but if you are producing a lot of milk, or more than your baby needs, you may feel full for longer. (See page 131.)

Blocked ducts – This is quite common and often recurs, so you need to familiarise yourself with my simple tips in order to prevent this happening and manage the situation effectively. When you know how to do this, this issue won't be a problem and you'll be able to resolve it quickly when it does occur. (See page 181.)

Low milk supply – As your storage capacity is reduced by your implant, you are more likely to feel 'full' and this can affect your production. So feed, feed and feed if you feel your supply is dropping.

Fast flow issues – With restricted storage capacity your milk flow will be fast and forceful to start with, which may give baby more wind. (See page 58 for winding tips.)

TIP

Breast surgery doesn't always mar breastfeeding. You won't know how much you can produce until you try – and you may just be surprised.

➜ Breast-reduction surgery

Breast-reduction surgery carries a risk of damaging glandular tissue and milk ducts. However, surgeons are more careful these days, so you should still be able to breastfeed your baby. At the very least, you will be able to combine breast- and bottle-feeds, but you may even be able to exclusively breastfeed. You won't know until you try!

Common challenges

Breast congestion – Some milk ducts can become damaged during surgery, making it difficult to transport milk. If this happens, certain parts of your breast will feel lumpy and may become inflamed.

Supplementation – You may not need to supplement baby with formula, but it is a good idea to decide which formula would be best for him before he arrives so that you have some to hand and feel better prepared, just in case.

TIP

Be aware that baby may need supplements, and if you use them do so without guilt.

37

When you know how to work with your individual breast shape and size, breastfeeding becomes more enjoyable. By understanding what is considered normal relating to your breast size, you can be better prepared rather than overwhelmed and caught off guard.

Feeling confident about knowing your breasts and how they can be used most productively for baby is important in deciding which hold and position is best to create the most effective and comfortable feed for your baby and for you. In the next chapter I will offer some options that work for all shapes and sizes.

CHAPTER 4

HOW TO HOLD AND POSITION YOUR BABY CORRECTLY
SETTING YOURSELF UP

The key to mastering a pain-free latch and comfortable feed is all down to how you hold and position your baby.

By holding him correctly, you will have more control when latching him on to the breast and he will be more relaxed and cooperative because he feels secure.

A good position ensures that you are both comfortable throughout the feed, regardless of how long it lasts. It also enables your baby to drain the entire breast efficiently with minimal effort, leading to an abundant, healthy milk supply and thriving baby.

This chapter is your first practical step forwards to getting breastfeeding right according to your unique mum-and-baby combination.

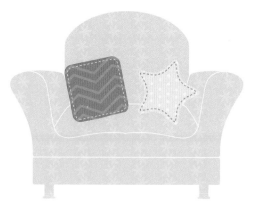

How to hold your baby comfortably

The closer your baby is tucked to your body, the easier it will be for him to scoop your breast up when he latches. Curl his lower arm around your side to cuddle your breast. Apart from keeping him very close to you, there are three additional key points to bear in mind.

1 Support your baby's entire body weight properly
If your baby is little, you can tuck his bottom into the crook of your arm. (*Fig. 1a*)

If he is bigger, use a rolled-up blanket or cushion to support his weight. (*Fig. 1b*)

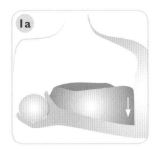 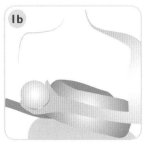

2 Place the ball of your hand on his upper back
This is vital for latching but also provides stability and a sense of security for baby. It is the most comfortable way for you to hold him and gives you good control. (*Fig. 2a & b*)

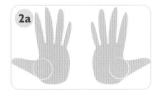 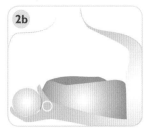

3 Support your baby's head comfortably
Splay your fingers open so that they spread over baby's entire cheek, to create an even spread of support. Ensure that there is nothing behind baby's head. (*Fig. 3*)

If baby turns his head down towards your fingers on his cheek, just move them back closer to his ears.

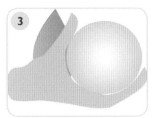

39

Troubleshooter tips

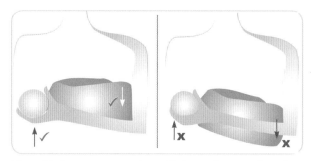

Keep his bottom up or he will slip and you will end up holding his head in a vice-like grip.

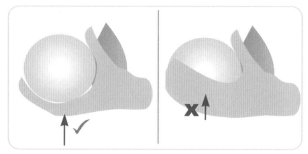

The back of baby's head should be free during the feed so that he can tilt his head back when latching and keep his nose unblocked to breathe.

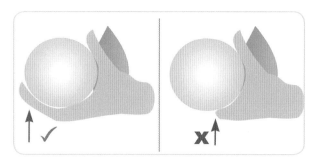

Use all your fingers to support baby's head, not just those on his jaw.

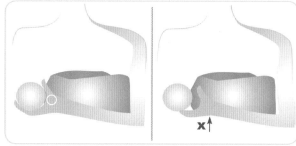

Your baby needs help to support his head, as his neck muscles are very weak to start with. Don't have your hand too far down his body or he will struggle to latch.

How to get into the right position

Once you know how to hold your baby, you need to get him into a good position in relation to your breast and nipple so that he can drain your entire breast effectively.

To achieve this, take these four points into consideration.

TIP

Your breast size determines how high up your body baby needs to be and whether or not you need a breastfeeding cushion.

1 **Your breast size**

Your breast size tells you how high up your body your baby needs to be in order to latch well and maintain a pain-free feed. By getting this right you can avoid sore nipples and breast lumps.

Small breasts (AA–D)
Your baby needs to be high enough to reach your breast. Consider using a breastfeeding cushion – preferably one that ties around your waist to stop it slipping away during the feed.

Medium breasts (DD–G)
You need to play around with different levels of support to get your baby to just the right height to reach your breast easily.

Large breasts (GG+)
You can try using something like a rolled-up blanket to start with.

Note
If using a breastfeeding cushion, be careful that baby is not higher than your nipple when your breast is at rest.

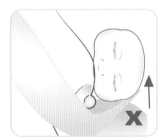

② The angle of your nipples

When you position your baby in line with your nipple angle, both his cheeks will touch your breast evenly once latched. This ensures that he drains the upper and lower halves of your breast evenly. Do this and your feeds will be effective and you'll be less likely to develop mastitis.

When your nipples point forward (*Fig. 1*), your baby comes directly on to your breast so that both his cheeks touch your breast evenly once he is latched (*Fig. 2*).

When your nipples point downward (*Fig. 3*), your baby comes on to the breast at an angle so that both his cheeks touch your breast evenly once he is latched (*Fig. 4*).

Note

You can lift your breast with a folded muslin cloth if you find positioning your baby tricky. (*Figs. 5&6*)

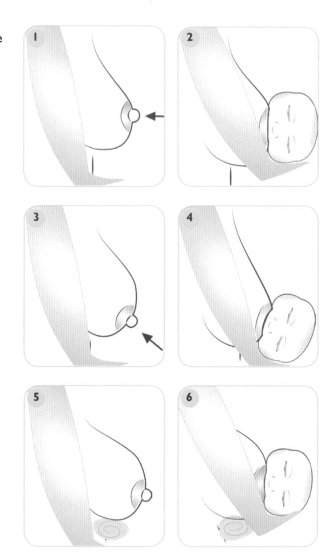

TIP

Run your finger along the underside of your breast to check that baby's lower cheek is flush with your breast.

③ Your milk flow

The position you feed in will increase or decrease your milk flow. You can manage your flow and baby's wind intake by making simple adjustments to your position (see page 47).

When you sit upright or lean slightly forward (*Fig. 1*), gravity increases milk flow to make it easier for baby to get milk with little effort. This is good for weak babies or if you have a slow milk flow.

When you lean right back (*Fig. 2*), gravity slows the flow of your milk by pulling it back into the breast, making it easier for baby to manage a forceful spray or oversupply.

④ Your birth story

You

Labour and birth can leave you feeling bruised and sore soon after birth. If your bottom is sore, sitting upright will be very uncomfortable. The same can be said if you have had a C-section. Don't feel pressured to sit upright; feed leaning back, lying down or even standing up. Try to find a position that is most comfortable for you while you are healing.

Your baby

During birth, your baby is squished and squashed as he makes his way into the world. He is supple and perfectly designed to undergo intense birth pressures but sometimes they will leave him feeling tight. Often his right side becomes more compressed and this can make feeding on your left breast tricky. Have a look at the slide-over position on page 50, which can make things easier. Also see page 51 for troubleshooting latching tips.

43

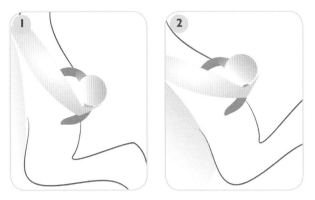

TIP

A tough delivery can lead to a bumpy breastfeeding start but it will get better. Don't beat yourself up if it's not as easy as you thought it would be.

Classic breastfeeding positions

↪ **The cross-cradle position**

This position is better for:

• mums with small- to medium-sized breasts
• mums learning to breastfeed
• mums who are able to sit upright comfortably
• mums who have a slow to moderate flow

1 Lift baby's bottom into the crook of your arm. His body should rest on top of your arm and his legs should be by your side. His lower arm is curled around your waist. (*Fig. 1*)

2 Place the soft ball of your hand on baby's upper back or upper spine. (*Fig. 2*)

3 Spread your fingers evenly across baby's lower cheek, so that you support his head and face evenly. When he gapes widely, bring your baby on to the breast by applying gentle pressure to his upper back with the ball of your hand. (*Fig. 3*)

4 Once you have latched baby on to your breast, support his bottom with a firm cushion and swap arms. When you swap arms to cradle him, replace the ball of your latching hand with the ball of your cradling hand so that there is nothing behind baby's head and you maintain gentle pressure on his upper back. (*Fig. 4*)

Left breast   Right breast

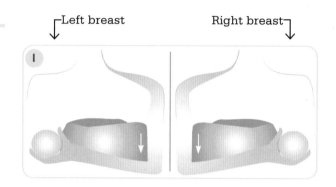

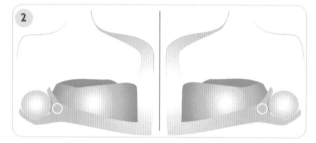

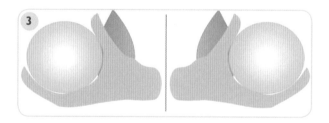

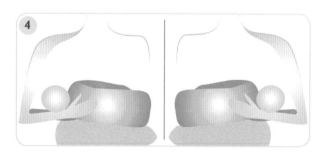

➙ The cradle position

This position is better for:
- mums with medium and large breasts
- mums with older babies
- mums with heavy or long babies
- babies who prefer to be cradled
- mums with a slow to moderate flow

① Support baby's body with a firm cushion so that he is at the right height and in line with your nipple. His lower arm should be curled around your waist. (*Fig. 1*)

② Place the ball of your hand on baby's upper back. (*Fig. 2*)

③ His head should be cradled in your wrist, with additional support from your thumb.

④ When baby gapes widely, bring his body quickly into the breast, applying gentle pressure with the ball of your hand.

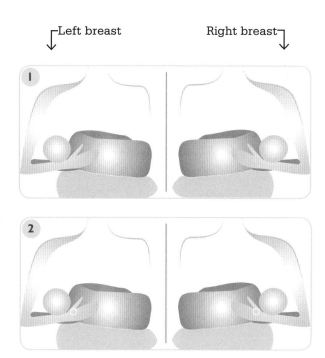

Left breast   Right breast

45

> **TIP**
>
> Be sure that your hand is in the right place or your baby's nose will make first contact with your breast and your latch will be painful.

↪ The underarm position

This position is better for:

• mums with large breasts
• mums who have had a C-section
• a baby who prefers to only feed from one side
• mums with twins
• mums with a slow flow

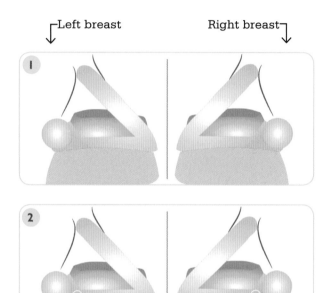

Left breast   Right breast

1 Support baby's body with a firm cushion so that he is at the right height and in line with your nipple. If you are supporting your back with cushions, ensure that they don't compromise his space. His lower arm should be curled around your waist. (*Fig. 1*)

2 Place the soft ball of your hand on baby's upper back. (*Fig. 2*)

3 Your fingers should evenly spread on baby's lower cheek and over his ear.

4 When he gapes widely, bring your baby on to the breast by applying gentle pressure to his upper back with the ball of your hand.

> *TIP*
>
> Lie your baby square on his side facing your breast if your nipples point forward. Roll your baby under your breast slightly if your nipples point downward.

Positions to moderate your supply

When you lean back, gravity pulls your milk back into your breast and slows down your flow. This is an easy way to help your baby cope with a fast and forceful let-down, as well as reducing the amount of wind baby swallows during the feed.

You can tweak common positions such as the cross-cradle and underarm positions when feeding out and about. At night or first thing in the morning when your supply is highest you can try feeding in the lying-down position.

➙ **Extended cross-cradle position**
This position is better for:
• mums with a fast flow or oversupply
• babies who have reflux

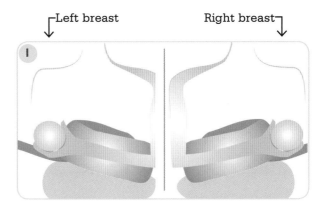

Latch your baby on to the breast using either the cradle or cross-cradle position. Once you are comfortable, lean right back. *(Fig. 1)*

Ensure that your lower back is well supported and that his position at the breast doesn't change when you lean back.

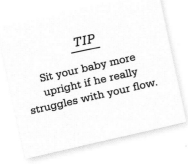

TIP

Sit your baby more upright if he really struggles with your flow.

47

➡ Extended underarm positions

These positions are better for:

- mums with fast flow
- mums with twins
- babies who have reflux
- babies who struggle with fast flow

TIP

Once baby has latched, you can support his weight with an additional cushion to take the pressure off your arm.

Facing mum

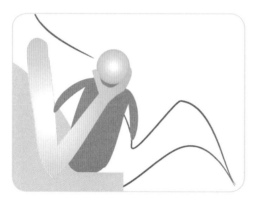

Facing the sofa

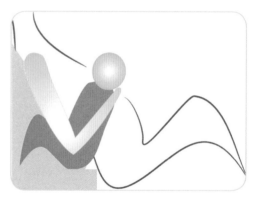

This version of the extended underarm position is good for mums who have small breasts and a small baby who is struggling to cope with fast and forceful let-downs.

Ensure that you lean right back to slow your flow, then sit baby upright, facing you. He'll come on to the breast from the side.

Use a cushion to lift him so that he can easily reach the breast, then support his back and head and latch him on to the breast.

This version of the extended underarm position is good for mums who have large breasts, a tall baby or a baby with a tongue-tie (see page 138).

Lift your breast with a rolled-up muslin, if you like.

Sit baby upright, facing the back of the couch, ensuring that you have created enough legroom for him by shuffling your bottom forward and using a good cushion for support.

Use a cushion to lift or raise baby so that he is able to reach the breast. Support his back with your arm and latch him on to the breast.

➜ The lying-down position

This position is better for:
• mums who have had a C-section
• mums with a fast flow
• babies who had assisted deliveries

Lie on your side with one arm under your head and your knees slightly bent.

Lie baby square on his side facing the breast, with his lower arm underneath the breast to raise it. Keep him close to you with his upper lip in line with your nipple.

Place your free hand on baby's upper back. When baby gapes, bring him on to the breast by applying gentle pressure to his upper back with your hand.

Once your baby has latched on to the breast, you can place a rolled-up muslin behind his back to keep him on his side and prevent him rolling back or away from the breast during the feed.

Tuck his bottom close to you to free his nose from your breast.

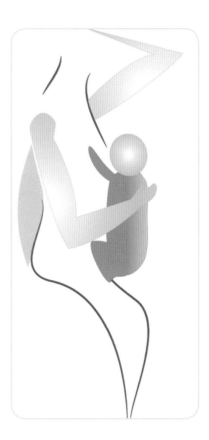

TIP

This is not a good position to use if your nipples are sore and baby doesn't do a wide mouth.

Many mums enjoy feeding like this for the late afternoon feed. It's a lovely way to catch up on some sleep yourself while your baby has an afternoon snooze too.

When feeding like this, ensure that your baby lies in the middle of the bed or close to the wall, with you on the outside edge.

49

↦ The slide-over position

This position is better for:
• babies with cranial tightness who prefer lying on one side

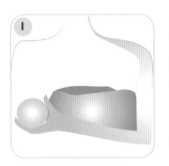

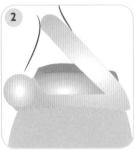

> *TIP*
>
> Ensure that you support baby's entire head to prevent him chomping your breast.

Your baby may feel uncomfortable when lying on one side and this makes latching difficult. In order to avoid unnecessary problems, keep baby comfortable and happy by laying him on his side when feeding on each breast.

To enable baby to feed from both sides, feed him in the cross-cradle position or across your lap on his preferred side. (*Fig. 1*)

Support his cheek with your fingers fanned open, so that there is not too much pressure on his lower jaw.

When feeding on the less-preferred breast, feed him in the underarm position so that he continues to lie on his comfortable side. (*Fig. 2*)

When you hold and position your baby in line with your anatomy, it feels good. You'll find that he is less flappy or unsettled and you will have good control. There are many variations of the key positions, so find or tweak one to suit your needs.

If baby is impatient for a feed you can alter your position to increase your flow, or you can adjust it to slow it down. Think outside the box when you are feeding – there are no restrictions – do what feels best for you and your baby. It is worth experimenting to get the right position, because when you find one that feels comfortable, latching baby on to the breast is quick and simple, as you'll see in the next chapter.

CHAPTER 5

HOW TO LATCH YOUR BABY
MAKING THE CONNECTION

This is where everything falls into place as you and your baby perfectly slot together like two pieces of a puzzle.

A good latch is built on to a great position, so if you hold your baby in a way that is comfortable for both of you and position him in line with your breast and nipple, all that's left to do is latch.

As your baby opens his mouth, you will give him a quick little hug to bring his body towards you. When you get it right, latching is an absolute dream and breastfeeding becomes a doddle.

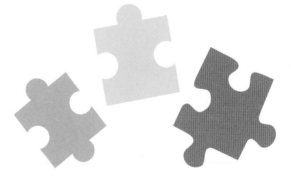

The nitty gritty of latching

As your baby comes on to the breast, a sequence of steps happens without you even noticing. The secret is to get baby's chin to indent your breast in the right place, so that your breast folds into his mouth without fuss.

➡ Start by lining baby's nose up with your nipple (*Fig. 1*), so that baby can scoop up as much areola close to his lower lip as possible. (*Fig. 2*)

➡ Bring him into the breast quickly, applying gentle pressure to his upper back so that his chin indents your breast. (*Fig. 3*)
    Your nipple just skims under his top lip and moves to the back of his mouth as his chin continues to indent your breast.

➡ Your areola lies on his tongue and your nipple is far back in his mouth. (*Fig. 4*)

➡ You will know right away that your latch is right as it won't hurt and you'll feel a tugging, rather than a biting sensation. Your baby will be calm and start suckling quite quickly to call his first let-down.

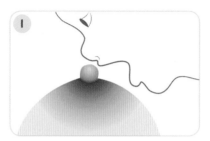

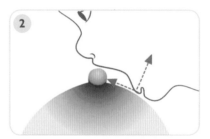

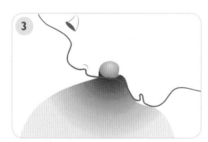

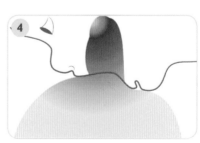

52

How to know if you're getting it right

Looking down at baby, you will see that his chin indents the breast and that his nose is free. (*Fig. 1*)

If his nose is too close to your breast, tuck his bottom closer to you and check that nothing is behind his head. (*Fig. 2*)

At the end of the feed, when your baby comes off the breast, you will see that the tip of your nipple is round like a hazelnut. (*Fig. 3*)

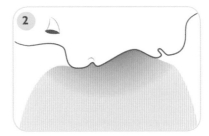

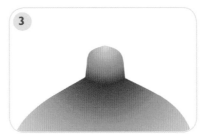

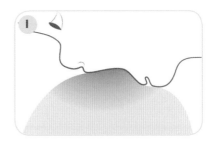

53

TUGGING OR BITING?

Once your baby has latched correctly, you should feel a tugging sensation.

If it feels like biting, you will know it's wrong and that baby's lower lip is too close to your nipple when latching.

Tugging is good. Biting is bad!

Latching techniques

In my practice, I advise mums to use variations of my top two troubleshooting techniques. If you are still finding latching tricky, try these for a more comfortable latch. However, before latching, make sure that you are holding and positioning your baby correctly.

→ Pinch and Pop technique (opposite)
This technique enables you to mould your breast into a graspable shape, making it easier for baby to get on to the breast quickly.

It is a good technique if you have:
- a full and firm breast
- a baby who is not latching well
- a baby who shuts his mouth early
- sore nipples that sting at the start of a feed

Your aim is to shape your breast into a breast sandwich in line with baby's smile, so that he can grasp and hold on to it with ease.

TIP

Your fingers should be in a 'V' for victory, not 'C' for can't latch as your breast is shaped perpendicular to his smile.

→ Brush and Clip technique (see page 56)
This technique is foolproof when done correctly. It is great for all mums and babies but may help you more if:
- your baby won't open his mouth
- your baby is sleepy
- you want him to get more areola
- your nipples are very sore and you need a foolproof technique

Your aim is to brush your baby's lower lip down using your areola edge and keep it pinned down so that you can quickly bring baby on to the breast before his mouth shuts.

A quick illustration. Pretend that your thumbnail is your nipple and your knuckle the edge of your areola.

Put your right thumb in a 'thumbs up' position and bend it down from the knuckle, so that it points away from you. Use your thumb knuckle to brush your lower lip down and open before popping your thumb into your mouth.

Mirror image of technique

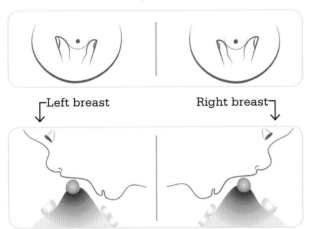

⌐Left breast   Right breast⌐

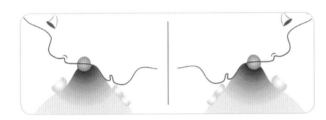

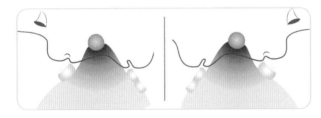

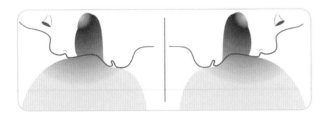

Pinch and Pop technique

1 Use thumb and index fingers to create a 'V' shape. Place your thumb and index finger at 3 o'clock and 9 o'clock, as far from the nipple as possible.

2 Pinch your thumb and index finger together to bunch up your breast and create a sandwich for him to latch on to.

3 Aim your nipple towards the roof of his mouth so that he has an off-centre latch.

4 Your breast will quickly fill his mouth and feel comfortable.

5 Once he has done a few stabilising sucks, carefully let go of the breast. If your breast moves downwards or to the side, move baby in the same direction to keep him latched effectively.

Mirror image of technique

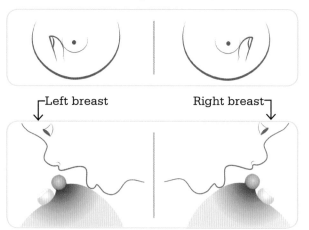

⌐Left breast   Right breast⌐

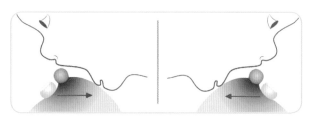

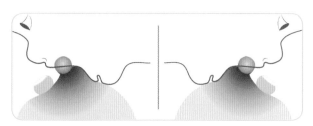

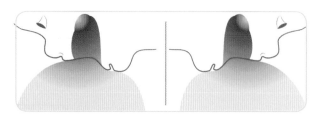

56

Brush and Clip technique

① Place your thumb on your areola on the outer side of your nipple. Push your thumb into your breast and pull it back a little so that your nipple points away from baby and the inner side of your areola bulges slightly.

② Line your baby up nose to nipple, so that his lower lip is close to your areola edge. It is important that baby gets more areola close to his lower lip for a comfortable latch and better feed.

③ With baby's lower lip on or near your inner areola edge, move your breast inwards and use your areola to coax baby's mouth open and curl his lower lip down.

④ Bring him on to the breast quickly by applying pressure to his upper back. As you bring baby on to the breast, your nipple will just skim under his top lip.

⑤ Once your baby has latched, remove your thumb. If your thumb gets in the way, just position it further away from the nipple when you next latch.

TOP TIPS FOR SUCCESSFUL LATCHING ON

Bring baby on to the breast quickly,
applying gentle pressure
to his upper back.

•

His chin should lead so that it
indents the breast and pulls
your nipple down.

•

He should have an off-centre
latch with his lower lip away from
the nipple base.

Use a latching technique if
he doesn't know what to do.

•

Check that his cheeks touch
the breast evenly.

•

If you feel biting and your nipple
is pinched at the end of the feed, your
latch is wrong. If you feel tugging
and your nipple is round at the end
of the feed, your latch is right.

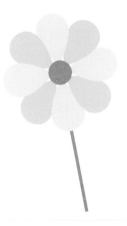

The better your baby is positioned and latched during feeding, the more milk and less air he will get during the feed. This is important, as reducing his wind intake where possible will help prevent trapped wind, which can and will make your baby feel very uncomfortable and lead to colicky episodes at the end of the day when you want him to feel most relaxed. If he does take in some wind, there are a few techniques that will help alleviate the problem, which I will explain in the next chapter.

CHAPTER 6

HOW TO WIND YOUR BABY
STRAIGHTFORWARD PRACTICAL KNOW-HOW

Winding is often the forgotten part of a breastfeed, but without it all the effort you put into getting positioning, latching and feeding right just goes out the window. The trick to winding is to keep baby calm, hold his back straight and get rid of swallowed air as soon as it goes in.

Where possible, reduce the amount of air he swallows during the feed. If you have a fast flow, change your feeding position to slow down your flow (see page 47). Don't be afraid to break a feed to wind your baby if you can hear him gulping and clicking at the breast.

Good things to know

↦ Manage your milk stream

If you have a lot of milk, you are likely to have a long milk stream, and this can lead to baby swallowing a lot of wind. The sooner you wind him after he has swallowed a bubble, the easier it is to get up that air. Monitor your baby's swallows and if he swallows more than 10 times before pausing, take him off your breast to allow him to catch his breath. The less air he swallows, the less wind you need to get up after the feed.

↦ Active winding (you are still and baby moves)

Active winding techniques are gentle baby-yoga-type movements that help baby to bring up stubborn burps. It is stimulating, so it can also be used to wake him up for feeding before you begin instead of a nappy change.

↦ Passive winding (you move and baby is still)

Passive winding techniques are calming and best used at the end of the feed when baby is full and you want to keep him calm. My Magic Hold on page 63 is pure gold and stops nine out of ten babies crying immediately!

↦ Start with the scoop hold and graduate to side-sitting hold.

When your baby is new and little, you'll feel more comfortable and confident if you hold him with both hands. This allows you to wind him without worrying about whether you are supporting his head properly.

Basic techniques

Once you have your baby in position, your winding possibilities are endless. There is no script, so just go with the flow, try a few things out and see how your baby responds. Remember to keep all movements slow and steady so that they feel like relaxing, gentle stretches to your baby.

↦ Pat or rub baby's back

Start right at the bottom and move upwards, straightening his back as you go. If you are using the scoop hold, lie him back and support him with one hand, patting him with the other.

↦ Bounce baby gently

Keep baby upright and jig your knee up and down quickly while supporting the back of baby's head. If you do this rhythmically you will find that he stops crying or calms down.

↦ Jig baby from right to left

Put your hand on baby's back, midway up, then jiggle your hand quickly to the left and right. You should see that this relaxes him and his shoulders jiggle right and left as your hand moves from side to side. Use the palm of your hand on his chest to apply gentle pressure to keep him in place and feel supported. This only works in the side-sitting hold.

How to hold your newborn

When your baby is new and little, you'll feel more comfortable and confident if you hold him with both hands. This allows you to wind him without worrying about whether or not you are supporting his head properly or choking him using the side-sitting hold.

↦ How to hold a newborn

The scoop hold is perfect to start with. Use both hands to support baby's body and the back of his head. The best bit about this technique is that you can keep eye contact with him and have a chat with him at the same time.

Scoop hold

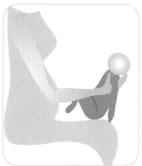

Sit your baby on your lap, close to your knees, facing you. Slip your fingers under baby's arms and use your fingertips to support the back of his head.

Use the palms of your hands to support baby's sides for more comfort and better control.

Active winding techniques for newborns

↦ Scoop corkscrew

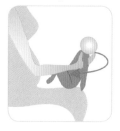

Starting with your baby upright, move his body clockwise in a circular movement while keeping his back nice and straight. Let him lean right back to stretch and then come forward right over his knees.

↦ Tipping teapot

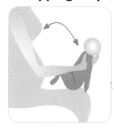

Start with your baby upright, then tip him back really slowly until he is almost lying flat. He may do a little stretch himself before you bring him back up to sitting position.

↦ Wind the bobbin up

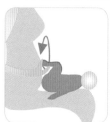

Lie baby on his back on your lap with his head near your knees and his bottom close to your stomach. Hook your thumbs behind his knees and gently bring his knees up and circle them. You can also hold his feet if it is easier.

Work with your baby. If he kicks back or stiffens up when using this technique, he probably has accumulated wind in his gut. Try another technique and come back to this one later.

How to hold your older baby

↪ **Side-sitting hold**

This is easier to do once you have had a bit of practice at holding a baby and you feel more confident. The trick here is to keep baby's back super straight.

Step 1

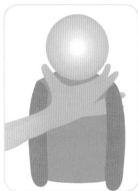

Place your palm on baby's chest with your thumb and index fingers on his cheeks, gently supporting his jaw line. Slide your ring and little fingers into baby's armpit. Use these to lift baby and straighten his back for better results.

Step 2

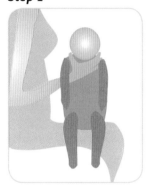

Sit baby on your outer thigh, midway between your hip and knee, and have the other leg ready to lift and support his back if he suddenly throws himself back.

61

Step 3

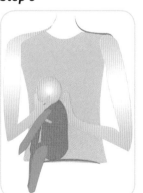

Use your free hand to pat or rub his back, or to support his head and upper body when you move him around or lie him down.

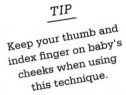

TIP

Keep your thumb and index finger on baby's cheeks when using this technique.

Active winding techniques for your older baby

↪ Corkscrew

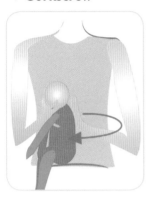

Keeping your front hand in the default position and supporting baby's back with your other hand, slowly lean baby back, then away from you, forward and towards you in a nice big corkscrew motion.

It can be quite an exaggerated move but do it slowly, so that your baby finds it relaxing and calming. If you do it too quickly, it is very likely that your little one will feel giddy and bring up his entire feed. Think of it as baby stretching or yoga.

↪ Tipping teapot

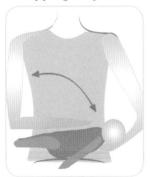

Ensure that you support the back of baby's head properly and tip him back slowly. Keep your leading hand in the default hold so that you can bring him back into the sitting position in one slow smooth movement.

↪ Wind the bobbin up

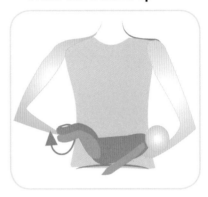

Lie baby on his back across your lap, as this is easier with a bigger baby, and support his head with one hand. Use the other hand to lift his legs and move them in a circular motion (clockwise).

You can also lift baby's legs and then drop them again or cycle them if he is really struggling with bottom wind. If baby is stiff, move to another hold and come back to this one again later.

TIP

You know your baby has winded enough when he is floppy and relaxed.

Passive winding techniques

This relaxes and winds him simultaneously, so it is great at the end of the feed when he is full and you want him to go to sleep.

↪ **Over the shoulder**

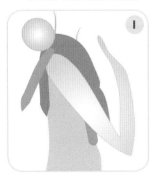

Scoop baby up, with your palms on his side and your fingers supporting the back of his head. Lift him over your shoulder then bring him down so that his armpits rest on your shoulder and he clips into place. Allow his back to stretch nicely or, if he is new, tuck his legs up like a little tree frog.

Use your outer hand to steady baby, so that he doesn't slip off your shoulder, and the other to pat his back.

You can also just hold him in position and then bounce by bending your knees while standing up, or while sitting on a Swiss ball or on the edge of your bed if you are too tired to stand.

↪ **The Magic Hold**

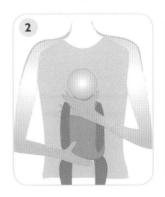 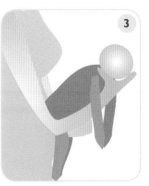

This is my signature hold, and when done correctly will stop nine out of ten babies crying instantly. (*Fig. 2*)

Support baby's cheeks and chest using the default hold (page 61) with one hand and cupping baby's tummy with your other hand. Sit baby's bottom on your belly button and tip him forward, keeping his back straight. Hold him in position and bounce from your knees. (*Fig. 3*)

You will know that you are doing this hold correctly when:
- your thumb and index finger are on baby's cheeks rather than on his neck
- baby's weight is supported by your tummy
- baby's chest relaxes into the palm of your hand
- you are jigging up and down
- baby is growing calmer and getting sleepy

63

↪ The Father's Hold

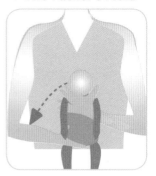 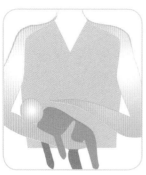

This hold is great for winding, going up and down stairs or just hanging out. It also gives you a free hand to answer the phone or the door.

To get to this position, sit baby against your front with him facing away from you and his back against you.

Slip your right hand over baby's right shoulder, over his front and between his legs. Hold on to his left leg for added safety.

Tip baby on to your right arm and get comfortable. Check that he has one arm on either side of your arm. This ensures that he is well balanced and safe.

With baby in place, you can now stand up and safely move around with him snugly tucked close to you. His head should rest on the fleshy bit of your forearm for most comfort.

You can use your free hand to pat or rub baby's back if he is windy or, if it is easier, you can just jig or bounce up and down as you would do if using the Magic Hold.

ESSENTIAL WINDING TIPS

There is no right or wrong way to wind your baby, just ways that suit you both.

•

You can reduce wind intake in the first instance by changing your feeding position to slow down your flow.

•

Wind baby during the feed if you hear him gulping or making a clicking noise.

•

Help him to relax first so that he is able to let go of trapped wind.

•

You have winded him enough when he is calm, floppy and relaxed.

You now have all the basic practical tools to get on with breastfeeding and make it a success. Breastfeeding is different for everyone, so don't worry if what you do is totally different to what your sister or best friend does. In the next chapter you will find everything you need to get you started with your baby on your own, unique breastfeeding journey.

PART 2:
BREASTFEEDING BABY

CHAPTER 7

YOUR FIRST FEEDS
HELLO BABY

Your first 24 hours with your newborn baby is a standalone experience, when everything feels very new and exciting. At some point during this time, take a moment to pause and soak up the miracle of birth, the experience of meeting your baby and the emotions you are feeling at becoming a mum. It is not an everyday occasion, so allow yourself to enjoy it.

Now is the time to put any pressures to one side and just feel your way through the first day. Rest, respond to your baby's cries and have as much skin-to-skin time as possible to reassure your newborn that you are close and there to keep him safe.

As your baby experiences full body contact with you he will become calm and feel settled and secure – which is such a lovely, gentle transition into a noisy, bright and cold world. Today, and for as long as you can, keep the outside world, with all its pressures, out of your baby bubble.

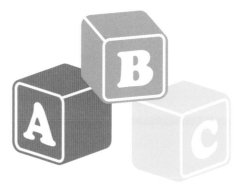

Day 0

➙ Your first breastfeed

Remind yourself that your body and your baby have been preparing for breastfeeding for months, so don't worry about needing to do anything special.

Lie back and put baby face down on to your stomach and just wait for all the puzzle pieces to come together. He may not start rooting immediately, but this is ok. Give him time to catch his breath, orientate himself and become interested in feeding. It will happen eventually.

Give him space to show you his moves as he crawls and wriggles upwards to find and latch on to your breast. He may take the scenic route, so give him some direction and use your arms to keep him from overshooting the nipple.

When he latches, let him feed until he is satisfied before offering the second breast. He may feel that he has had enough or he may decide to have some from the second side as well.

➙ After the first feed

Your baby may want to sleep for a few hours, but thereafter it is worth offering him some colostrum every four to five hours. Wake him by doing gentle winding (see page 60) or a nappy change if he is very sleepy. Alternatively, you can just put him on to your chest and he'll soon rouse.

When you feed your baby little and often he gets drip-fed small portions of colostrum frequently. This stimulates your production and activates hormone receptor cells, which are most sensitive in the first three days (see page 19).

Feeding little and often also stops him from becoming too hungry to focus on latching properly.

If he cries as soon as you put him down, he is probably just unsure of his new surroundings and wants to be with you. Keep him close to you or get your husband to hold him skin to skin while you rest.

➙ Contraction pains

Oxytocin is responsible for contractions during labour as well as contracting muscles around your milk sacs to create a let-down. When your baby breastfeeds, your body releases oxytocin and all the muscles affected by oxytocin contract.

As your uterus contracts, you'll have sharp period-type pains, but this only lasts for a couple of days. It is important for your uterus to contract back to its pre-pregnancy size and shape as well as to slow down any post-birth bleeding. You can place a hot water bottle on your bump pre and post feeds for added comfort.

⇢ Feeding positions

Depending on what your labour and delivery were like, you may feel more comfortable in one particular position – even if it is not your favoured position (see page 46). Do what works for you at the time. As everything calms down and you feel better, you can rejig your position and get on with breastfeeding as you had originally planned.

If you had an assisted birth (ventouse or forceps) or a C-section, you may find feeding in a version of the lying-down position easiest (see page 49).

⇢ Sleepy baby

New babies love to snuggle into you during the feed. If your baby is very sleepy and not feeding, compress your breast to keep your colostrum flowing and baby feeding (see page 21).

⇢ Conflicting advice

Don't be surprised if you get different suggestions and advice from every midwife that comes to see you. They are all trying to help out but are not breastfeeding specialists. Trust your instincts and follow the gentle guidelines in this book.

TIP

Give your baby as much time as he needs to get breastfeeding right. There is NO rush.

↪ Good things to know

Skin to skin

By keeping baby skin to skin, you reduce his stress hormones and encourage the release of endorphins – so you are his medicine! As your body also releases endorphins when baby is skin to skin with you, he is your medicine too. Do as much skin to skin as possible.

Breast compression

When your baby is little and in a hurry for food, a slow flow is frustrating. You can increase milk flow and help baby get as much milk for minimal effort by compressing your breast with a flat hand (see page 21).

Switch-nursing

You can move back and forth between both breasts, using compression for better flow, until he is full and satisfied. This is an easy way for him to get enough colostrum in a short feed (see page 163).

Pinch and Pop technique

Assisted births can make baby feel quite tight and sore, especially if he was not in a great position in the womb, was turned or ended up arriving via an emergency C-section. You don't have any control over that but you can help him by shaping your breast, in line with his smile, to help him get on to the breast (see page 54).

Hand-expressing

You can express droplets of colostrum and rub this on to your baby's gums and tongue if he is not latching on. Remember his stomach is tiny and colostrum is potent so even a couple of drops will stabilise his blood sugar levels. See page 98 for how to do it.

Night feeds

Most babies are happy to sleep for a bit longer on the first night, giving you the opportunity to catch your breath. If your baby is awake all night and doesn't give you a second's break, bring your daytime feeds as close together as possible so that he gets more calories during the day.

69

> *TIP*
>
> Feed your baby every two to three hours from the start of one feed to the start of the next, day and night, until day 5.

MONITOR BABY'S POOS

Your baby's poos give you a clear indication of how much milk he is getting and whether that is enough. When he gets what he needs his poos start as black and become lighter each day until, by day 10, they are yellow.

The number of 50p-size poos he does each day will show you what he is getting in volume. Each day we expect to see the number of poos increase by one, starting on day 1, until we get to day 8 and he is doing eight poos, usually halfway through the feed. He will continue to do a poo at each feed until week 6.

Some babies are natural overachievers and get ahead of their poo spectrum, skip a few colours and end up at yellow poos a lot earlier. This is not a problem; it shows you that your baby is getting more than enough milk and what you are doing is perfect.

If your baby's poos are slow to change, it is the first sign that you need to get more milk into him. You want to get to yellow poos as quickly as possible, then once they are yellow they should stay yellow going forward.

Here's a rough idea of what to expect in the first 10 days:

DAY 0 One black poo
DAY 1 One black poo
DAY 2 Two black poos

DAY 7 Seven orange poos
DAY 8 Eight orange poos

DAY 3 Three spinach-green poos
DAY 4 Four spinach-green poos

DAY 9 Eight yellow poos
DAY 10 Eight yellow poos

DAY 5 Five dark brown poos
DAY 6 Six dark brown poos

Day 1

You have made it through the first 24 hours and breastfeeds can still feel a bit intense as you and baby are learning what to do. Your baby is 24 hours old, so officially one day old. You may be experiencing similar challenges to yesterday, so follow the same troubleshooters and give baby a chance to find his feet.

➺ Cave baby instincts

Your baby is programmed to sleep all day and feed all night. In the cavemen days you would be vulnerable to being eaten during the day when the men were out hunting, which is why your baby sleeps and your supply is lowest between 1 and 4pm. At night, you'd be protected by the menfolk so that you and baby could co-sleep and feed all night when your supply is at its peak.

➺ Feeding

To help baby turn his days and nights around, feed him often, roughly every three to four hours, calculating feeds from the start of one feed to the start of the next.

Continue to offer baby both sides so that he gets plenty of colostrum. Your feeds may take an hour at this stage. It doesn't matter how long they take, provided he gets enough and the feeds are enjoyable. If you feel that the feeds are taking a tad too long, use breast compression to speed them up a smidge.

➺ Poos

His poos are still black and on day 1 and you want to see at least one poo the size of a 50p coin. If he has not done a poo today but did a massive one yesterday, he has probably cleared his entire digestive tract, so look out for one tomorrow.

➺ Night feeds

If you had a rough night, get baby on to your chest and feeding at least every two to three hours, calculating feeds from start to start, or more frequently if he asks. The more your baby feeds during the day, the better he will sleep at night.

➺ Nipple shields

Where possible, I try not to introduce artificial teats before breastfeeding is going well, but nipple shields can really help your baby get your milk. It's not ideal but still a viable option to get your baby feeding from your breast. If your baby is not getting on to the breast, is crying, expending energy and you are worried about him, you can use nipple shields to give him something firm to latch on to. It will enable him to get your colostrum and avoid the need for formula (see page 180).

Every day things will get a little easier, just stick with it and keep baby close for now.

If you had a rough night, do more skin to skin with baby today. Get him on to your chest every three hours or so.

Day 2

It is normal for breastfeeding to feel stressful and erratic in the early days. It's not easy to feel relaxed when you aren't sure what is going on or what is meant to be happening and everyone tells you something different. The only person who really matters is the little person in your arms. If he is happy then you are doing fine. Keep him close to you so that you can get to know him and his needs really well as soon as possible.

⇢ Feeding

Continue to feed at least three-hourly to start with, offering both sides at each feed. You can switch freely between both breasts and use breast compression to keep colostrum flowing.

⇢ Poos

Poos are still expected to be black today and you want to see at least two small poos (see page 70). If they are turning dark green, you know that your baby is ahead of the curve and getting more colostrum than he needs.

⇢ Troubleshooting common challenges
Soothe your nipples

Your nipples may be a bit sensitive from all your breastfeeding but they shouldn't be cracked or bleeding. If they are, it tells you that something is wrong. It may be your positioning or latching but it could also just be down to a tricky birth (see page 135).

Express droplets of colostrum and rub them into your nipples after feeds to soothe them. You can also wear hydrogel breast discs to rehydrate and calm them between feeds (see page 182).

Nipple shields

If your nipples are very sore, cracked or bleeding, try using nipple shields for a few feeds to give your nipples a rest (see page 180).

Urates

Red or orange crystals in baby's nappy are called urates. They are pretty common in the early days when your baby doesn't get much fluid. It can be a sign of dehydration if the crystals become darker, but if they become lighter, you know that things are going the right way.

Poos

If your baby hasn't had a poo for over 24 hours you need to change your feeding pattern and offer baby the breast more often. If you are already doing that, you had a C-section, your nipples are sore or you have had breast-reduction surgery, you may need to offer him some formula.

Formula top ups

Your baby is now two days old so he will need around 20ml per three-hourly feed. If he is not having bowel movements, offer him formula at each feed until he does, to ensure that he doesn't lose too much weight or become too jaundiced.

The best way to offer formula is to:
• Start with 5ml to give him energy and take the edge off his hunger,
• Offer him both breasts, switching when he is not swallowing,
• Compress to keep milk flowing,
• Then finish with another 5 to 10ml of formula if needed.
• It's easier to use ready-made formula at this stage.

Tomorrow will be better. Don't worry if you have to give baby bits of formula to satisfy him, just keep feeding every three hours to stimulate your breasts. Use the formula to give him the energy to do a better job at the breast. Many mums use a bit of formula to keep breastfeeding going until their milk comes in and then they drop it (see page 107 for bottle-feeding tips).

TIP

A bit of formula if needed in the beginning is better than no breastfeeding in the end.

Day 3

Changes to breastfeeding are becoming more noticeable. You will have more volume at each feed, so baby should begin to settle better after feeds.

↝ Breasts
Your breasts may start feeling fuller, heavier and firmer to the touch if baby has been feeding well and often. This is a good sign and tells you that your milk is 'coming in'. Soon he will be flooded with transitional milk and you will see the 'milk-drunk look' that everyone talks about.

↝ Feeding
Continue to offer both breasts three-hourly, switching between them as necessary and using compression to make the feeds easier for baby. It's fine to feed sooner if baby is hungry; just go with the flow and try to feed more during the day if your nights are still active.

↝ Poos
Baby's poos should be turning a spinach-green now and you want to see three small poos over the course of the day. If his poos are already brown, orange or yellow, you know that he is getting enough colostrum. If they are slow to change colour, you need to feed more or top up until your milk comes in properly.

> *TIP*
> Breast-milk poos are very runny because your milk is so easily absorbed that there is very little wasted. Poos should be runny and yellow. This is not diarrhoea.

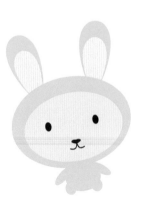

➜ **Troubleshooting challenges**

Milk

If you had a C-section or lost a lot of blood during delivery, your milk may come in later than day 3, leaving baby hungry. Feed your baby three-hourly and top up if you need to.

Be kind to yourself; Rome wasn't built in a day and certainly not by men immediately post-birth, so if you need to top up, do it. It is not failure and may well be the one thing that saves breastfeeding long term.

Tiredness

Nothing prepares you for the intensity of having a baby and how little sleep you will have. Sleep as much as possible during the day when baby sleeps. Just forget about housework, chores or anything non-baby-related for now. It will get easier, but until then, don't try to be a superwoman or continue life as you did pre-baby – you will just run yourself into the ground.

Maternity help

If you are on your knees at this point, get in some maternity help just to get you over the bump by catching up on some sleep and teaching you some key skills to make everything easy. My maternity nurses are a dream. (See Miskin Maternity on page 185.)

Food

The hours flurry by and you don't even notice when you miss meals as you are so consumed with life as a full-time mum, but you need to eat regularly and drink water with each feed. Support your body as it recovers from months of broken sleep, a labour, birth and a new full-on role of providing enough milk for your baby.

You will have a real sense of relief when your milk 'comes in', but it can bring about some challenges. I will cover these in a later chapter, but if you need some tips for engorgement see page 131.

Continue to monitor your baby's poos each day and check that they are tracking the poo spectrum outlined on page 70. Apart from weight gain, this is the only way to gauge how much milk your baby is getting at each feed.

Weight gain is less helpful in the first week, as your baby is expected to lose about 10 per cent of his birth weight by day 5 before he begins to gain weight regularly. We'll look at feeding in a bit more detail in the next chapter.

You are on the brink of a whole new experience. When your milk 'comes in', breastfeeding becomes so much easier. You have made it through the toughest bit and if you can do that, you can go all the way.

CHAPTER 8

HOW TO BREASTFEED IN THE FIRST THREE MONTHS
GETTING BREASTFEEDING RIGHT FOR YOU

Once your milk comes in and you have dealt with any engorgement issues, breastfeeding becomes easier because you feel confident that your baby is getting more milk. Provided your nipples are not damaged, you should find that you and baby start to carve out a more predictable feeding pattern.

Breastfeeding will become more predictable as your baby gets the hang of it. If your baby doesn't fall into a natural feeding pattern himself and feeding becomes stressful for both of you, follow a gentle three-hourly feeding rhythm, as this usually works for most babies. However, as all babies are different, your little one may prefer to feed more or less frequently.

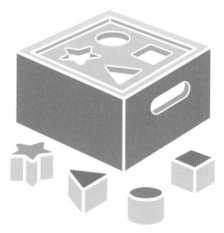

Day 4 to week 12

If you are not sure what sort of pattern your baby is on or what to do, start by noting down your goals as well as baby's needs.

Your goals	Baby's needs
Good effective feeds ⟶	Good weight gain
Healthy milk supply ⟶	Good positioning
Good sleep habits ⟶	Good winding

You can see that they all go hand in hand and that you and baby ultimately want the same things. This can get lost in translation when breastfeeding doesn't go smoothly. You may even feel that baby is working against you, but he isn't.

↪ Effective feeds and good weight gain

When your baby is able to access milk easily for little effort, he doesn't burn unnecessary calories, nor does he need to hang out at the breast for hours on end, as he gets what he needs in good time.

↪ Healthy milk supply and good positioning

You maximise glandular function and breast drainage when baby is positioned well, as he drains your entire breast effectively.

↪ Good winding helps a baby sleep well

If your baby gets enough milk during the day, there is no reason for him not to sleep well, other than the discomfort trapped wind causes. So if you get rid of this during the day, your nights will be much smoother.

How to know that he is getting enough

A good place to start is with weight gain and what's expected. This, along with monitoring output, is the only way to be sure that your baby is getting enough milk.

↪ Lost birth weight

By day 5, your baby will be at his lowest weight, having lost around 10 per cent of his birth weight, although it is likely to be less if feeds have been going well. You want to see that once baby has hit his lowest weight he starts gaining between 20g and 30g each day.

You will have two visits from the community midwives, who will weigh your baby before discharging you. Thereafter, you can have baby weighed once a week at the baby clinic held at your GP's practice.

↪ Regular weight gain

Once your baby has regained his lost birth weight (usually before week 3), he will gain steady increments each week. Tweak your feeding pattern to stabilise his weight gain.

To increase your baby's milk intake and weight gain, you can feed from both sides multiple times during the feed. You can move back and forth between both breasts, switching over to the other side when baby is not swallowing even though you are compressing the breast. This method of feeding is called switch-nursing.

Assessing your baby's weight gain at a glance

Less than 100g/3oz per week	Roughly 210g/7oz per week	More than 350g/12oz per week
Feed more frequently	Keep feeding as you are	Reduce frequency of feeds
Offer both sides at each feed	Monitor baby's weight gain	Feed when baby is hungry
Switch-nurse (R-L-R-L-R-L)		Offer one side per feed
Compress and top up if needed		Consider block feeding (see page 167)

→ Feeding patterns and routines

You can follow baby's lead and feed him when he asks for milk or you can begin to create structure to your day. Either approach is fine provided it is sustainable and baby is gaining weight well. Always offer a two-part feed (see page 82).

→ Bottle-feeds

If your baby doesn't feed well, you can express and bottle-feed expressed breast milk before introducing formula. You are more likely to get back to exclusive breastfeeding if you maintain a good supply.

On the next few pages I have outlined how feeding patterns typically progress for different breast and baby combinations. These are based on storage capacity and baby's milestones. They are just guidelines, though; so don't worry if your baby does something different.

TIP

Feed 2–3 hourly during the day and leave your baby to wake for feeds at night once he has regained his birth weight.

How to feed according to your breast and baby's size

→ **Breastfeeding combinations for small-breasted mums**

Small-breasted mums (AA–D)	Small baby (6lbs/2.5kg)	Average baby (8lbs/3.5kg)	Large baby (10lbs/4.5kg)
Weeks 0–1	2 breasts 2-hourly	3 breasts 2–3-hourly	4 breasts 2–3-hourly
Weeks 1–3	1–2 breasts 2–3-hourly	1–2 breasts 2–3-hourly	2 breasts 3-hourly
Week 3 (growth spurt)	1–2 breasts 2-hourly	2 breasts 2–3-hourly	3 breasts 2-hourly
Week 5 (growth spurt)	2–3 breasts 1–2-hourly	3 breasts 2–3-hourly	4 breasts 1–2-hourly
Week 6 and after	2–3 breasts 3-hourly	3–4 breasts 3-hourly	4+ breasts 3-hourly

Feed from both sides at each feed to get your supply established as quickly as possible. As your supply increases, your baby may refuse the second side, however this is more likely if he is small.

Monitor baby's output and weight gain regularly. Calculate his average daily gain, as this is the best way to assess how well you are meeting his needs.

• Older and bigger babies can be impatient when waiting for let-downs, so feel free to switch back and forth between the breasts during the feed.
• Breast compression is essential to keep the milk flowing.
• Provided baby's poos are yellow, you know that he is getting enough creamy milk at each feed.
• Once your baby is feeding three-hourly on a regular basis, see page 114 for suggestions on creating a routine.

→ **Breastfeeding combinations for medium-breasted mums**

Medium-breasted mums (DD–G)	Small baby (6lbs/2.5kg)	Average baby (8lbs/3.5kg)	Large baby (10lbs/4.5kg)
Weeks 0–1	1–2 breasts 2–3-hourly	2 breasts 2–3-hourly	2–3 breasts 2–3-hourly
Weeks 1–3	1 breast 2–3-hourly	1.5 breasts 2–3-hourly	2 breasts 2–3-hourly
Week 3 (growth spurt)	1.5 breasts 2-hourly	2 breasts 2–3-hourly	3 breasts 2-hourly
Week 5 (growth spurt)	2 breasts 2-hourly	3 breasts 2–3-hourly	4 breasts 2-hourly
Week 6 and after	1–2 breasts 3-hourly	2 breasts 3–4-hourly	2–3 breasts 3–4-hourly

Your morning feeds are likely to be short and effective and your afternoon feeds longer. This is fine and doesn't mean that your supply is 'running out'. Your baby is just feeding according to the peak and dip of your milk supply (see page 24).

• Ensure that you feed from both breasts at every feed by the second growth spurt to avoid developing an oversupply.
• Use breast compression conservatively towards the end of the feed when baby is full and sleepy to ensure he gets a full feed.
• Monitor baby's poos to check that he is getting enough creamy milk at each feed (see page 70).
• Once your baby is feeding three-hourly on a regular basis, see page 114 for routine suggestions.

➜ Breastfeeding combinations for large-breasted mums

Large-breasted mums (GG+)	Small baby (6lbs/2.5kg)	Average baby (8lbs/3.5kg)	Large baby (10lbs/4.5kg)
Weeks 0–1	1 breast 2-hourly	1.5 breasts 2–3-hourly	2 breasts 2–3-hourly
Weeks 1–3	1 breast 2–3-hourly	1.5 breasts 3-hourly	2 breasts 3-hourly
Week 3 (growth spurt)	1.5 breasts 2-hourly	2 breasts 2–3-hourly	2 breasts 2–3-hourlyy
Week 5 (growth spurt)	1–2 breasts 2–3-hourly	2–3 breasts 2–3-hourly	2–3 breasts 2–3-hourly
Week 6 and after	1–2 breasts 3-hourly	2 breasts 3–4-hourly	2–3 breasts 3–4-hourly

Always offer the first side twice before offering the second side in a feed. Bigger babies often prefer to feed every four hours as they have a larger stomach capacity. This is fine if your baby is gaining enough weight and doing plenty of wet and dirty nappies.

• Wind and nappy change mid-feed (during the day) to help baby feed efficiently and get what he needs.
• Use breast compression conservatively to keep baby interested and awake during feeds.
• Be aware that some large breasts have less glandular tissue and more fatty tissue. In these cases either follow the medium- or small-breast feeding patterns to ensure that baby gains enough weight. (See page 33.)
• Once your baby is feeding three-hourly on a regular basis, see page 114 for routine suggestions.

Length of feeds

On average, babies feed for 15–50 minutes per feed, but rather than focusing on how long your baby feeds for, monitor how frequently he swallows. Just as you can gulp down a large glass of water in a few seconds or sip on it for ages, your baby can drink milk very quickly or feed at a leisurely pace.

→ Two-part feed

- On average your baby will feed for 10–20 minutes before he does a poo and becomes sleepy.
- Wind him and change his nappy to wake him up and get him ready for a bit more milk. This allows the milk in his stomach to move into his gut.
- Feed him for another 10–20 minutes to refill his stomach.
- Do a quick bit of winding over your shoulder before you pop him down with a full stomach and gut.
- If you only do the first bit, he will be awake within 20 minutes of being put down for his 'second half'.

TIP

Your breast size will determine whether you feed from one or two sides before winding and nappy changing.

Milestones and challenges

→ Growth spurts

Your baby boosts your supply at certain points to ensure that it meets his growing needs. He does this by feeding more frequently for a couple of days at around weeks 3 and 5. We call these 'feeding frenzies' growth spurts.

The more frequently he feeds, the more your breasts are stimulated, which increases your supply. It is exhausting but very normal and over quickly if you allow baby free access to both breasts.

→ Possetting (bringing up milk)

Normal possetting happens infrequently and the volume your baby brings up is no more than a tablespoon or so. If baby has overfed, what he brings up will be clear and looks just like milk. If it is wind- or burp-driven, the milk will have curdled bits. This shows that you need to wind sooner into the feed. Normal possets come up in one wave and baby usually seems more comfortable afterwards.

→ Colic

The word colic is used loosely for babies who seem fussy after feeds and cry for 'no reason' for at least three hours each night. The most common culprit is trapped wind that accumulates throughout the day and keeps baby in a state of discomfort.

Colic is usually more noticeable after the first growth spurt at 3 weeks. This is probably due to your supply increasing and baby swallowing more air. By winding your baby diligently and allowing him space to settle between feeds, you should find this less of a problem. (See winding aids on page 184.)

Crying incessantly at the end of the day is more likely to be due to a combination of trapped wind and overtiredness. Look at the routines on page 117 and try to introduce a bit of structure to help get baby into some sort of feeding and sleeping pattern.

At around 3 weeks the muscles in your baby's gut start to contract in a wave-like motion to move waste along rather than be reliant on milk coming in. As this is new, the muscles need to learn to work together.

Until they do, it can feel like intermittent, isolated cramps, which is uncomfortable for baby. This can add to the colic theory but is actually just developmental. Make an appointment with a cranial osteopath, who can help with digestion.

→ Reflux

It is normal for babies and adults to reflux roughly 50 to 100 times a day. Babies bring up more food as their oesophagus is short in relation to their body, so bringing up milk is not a sign of something terrible.

Often reflux is exacerbated by trapped wind as the milk rides on top of a bubble and baby brings both up at the same time. Moderate your flow by changing your position to start with (see page 48).

Trapped wind or acid reflux

Baby's reaction to bringing up milk is the key factor to determining whether he has acid reflux or just bad wind. If your baby seems better, happier and calmer after bringing up milk, you can reassure yourself that it is just bad wind.

Your baby will scream the place down if he brings up milk and acid. This is when you need to get to your GP and discuss your options.

Silent reflux

When your baby has silent reflux, the milk and acid come into his oesophagus but not all the way out. It's like a phantom reflux. You will notice that your baby looks uncomfortable and starts to cry before swallowing down milk that has come up, after which he cries desperately.

You need to keep a diary of all your baby's symptoms and then go to your GP for a care plan and medication, if needed. Make an appointment there and then to come back and see your GP in seven days to assess the treatment plan. Don't let it drag on for weeks or months – it needs to get sorted.

➙ Pyloric stenosis

The defining difference between reflux and pyloric stenosis is that with pyloric stenosis the milk comes up in waves rather than just as a blip. You will notice this if your baby's pyloric valve (the one at the bottom of his stomach) is too tight and doesn't allow the milk out of baby's stomach. Baby thinks he is overfull and his stomach contracts to bring up 'excess' milk, which happens to be the entire feed.

Feed little and often so that his stomach doesn't overfill, and visit your GP. He will feel baby's stomach for a little 'knot' to confirm the diagnosis. Sometimes baby may need a surgical procedure to solve the problem, but altering feeds is usually all it takes to make things better.

➙ Awake time

Your baby will be able to stay awake for roughly one and a half hours now before becoming sleepy and tired. He may only be awake for a feed to start with but, as his feeds get shorter, he will have more awake time between feeds.

➙ Poos

As your baby gets older and bigger, his gut increases in length and this provides more storage capacity for waste. Around weeks 5 to 7, you'll notice that your baby poos less frequently, seems constipated and very unsettled. This is a normal developmental milestone.

What happens is that, as your baby has more space in his gut for the tiny amount of waste, gas builds in his gut and makes him feel uncomfortable. This is new to him as before he would be able to shift it, but now that there is more room in his gut for waste, it stays inside longer.

Use your winding techniques, focusing on 'Wind the bobbin up (see page 60) and moving his legs up to his chest. When you do a nappy change, have some nice hot water to hand to soak a cotton wool ball in and pop this on to his bottom. The moist heat from the cotton wool and gentle pressure will help him relax his anus and release excess wind. If your baby is struggling you can also offer him a few sips of cooled boiled water to help him do a poo.

TIP

Your baby will continue to do clear wees if he is getting enough milk, even if his poos are missing in action.

Troubleshooting challenges

➻ Reduce wind intake

Either wind your baby more frequently during the feed or change your feeding position to slow down your flow. If you can't find a position that works, try using nipple shields to moderate milk flow or feed baby sooner, before he is overly hungry. You can also reduce your supply (see page 169).

➻ Winding aids

While these are safe to use, don't use them if you think that your baby has acid reflux as it can make things worse. Instead, keep baby upright for at least 30 minutes after a feed or carry him upright in a sling, so that you can get on with other bits and bobs. You can raise the head of his Moses basket by placing sturdy books under the head of his bed, so that his head is higher than his bottom.

➻ Allergies

Reflux can be exacerbated by sensitivities and allergies to foods in your diet or foods that you have in excess. If there are any sensitivities in your family to certain foods, cut those out of your diet for at least two weeks before slowly introducing them again. Common foods to consider include dairy, soy, eggs, citrus and wheat. If you aren't sure where to start, ask your GP or get a referral to a paediatric allergist who will guide you.

➻ Slimy spinach-green poos

Slime or clear mucus in baby's poos tell you that his gut is irritated by something you are eating. If you are taking meds or antibiotics, this could also be making baby feel irritable and contributing to all of the above issues.

Green poos are also an indicator that baby is not getting as much cream as he could or should be, so if this is a standalone symptom, have a look at the oversupply chapter in the managing challenges section on page 166, as well as Colief drops on page 184.

Breastfeeding is different for all mums and babies, so please don't feel pressured to fit into a set pattern. You'll find what works for you by process of trial and error but as long as you keep looking at the big picture and not just one aspect of breastfeeding, it will all fall into place.

It is normal to run into some challenges when learning any new skill, so have a look at the troubleshooting chapters later in this book as and when you need to. Refresh your memory with the key elements of positioning and latching, too, because these change as your baby gets bigger and heavier.

Your baby is now growing and you will be beginning to establish a routine together. The next few months are all change again, as baby continues to develop, grow and be more active. The next chapter will take you through what to expect as your baby reaches three months old.

CHAPTER 9

HOW TO BREASTFEED BEYOND THREE MONTHS
KEEPING ABREAST

In the first three months of his life your baby develops at an alarming rate. He needs lots of calories to ensure he can grow stronger, and your supply matches his needs. It is teamwork – he boosts your supply by initiating growth spurts and you do all you can to maintain a good supply.

In the second three-month period, everything slows down. Your feeds will gradually become shorter and you'll have longer gaps between them. If your baby hasn't already carved out some sort of routine, he will start to fall into a recognisable pattern now, and this should include longer stretches of sleep at night.

Pulling off the breast to have a chat, look around or play is part and parcel of breastfeeding in the second three-month period. Your baby doesn't grow at the same pace as he did in the first three months. He is not as ravenous but instead more interested in communicating.

Changes continue to be subtle and you may not notice them until you look back over a week or two. In this chapter we'll look at common developments and challenges for each month.

Breastfeeding a three-month-old

At three months your baby has a good sense of his surroundings. He is strong enough to hold his head up, look around and engage with you. His cooing, gurgling and smiles brighten your day but when this constantly happens during feeds, it can be a tad frustrating, particularly when feeding in public.

As your baby's feeds become shorter, you may worry about how much he is getting at each feed and whether or not you should encourage him to feed for longer.

The only way to know that he is getting enough is to loosely monitor his weight gain.

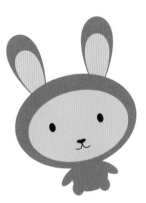

➻ Regular weight gain

Your baby will double his birth weight between four and six months. If he is close to doubling his birth weight already, loosely monitor his weight gain and closely monitor sleep patterns at night. If he gets what he needs during the day, he will sleep well at night.

For babies who are a long way off doubling their birth weight I would suggest that you calculate how much baby should gain each week and then find a way to achieve that.

Here's how you do it:
• Double baby's birth weight, so that you have an idea of what he should be weighing by week 24.
• Subtract his current weight from his doubled weight to see how much he needs to gain.
• Now subtract his current age in weeks from 24 to tell you how many weeks he has to gain the remaining weight.

For example:
Birth weight 3kg x 2 = 6kg by week 24
Current weight 4.5kg at 14 weeks
Your baby needs to gain 1.5kg in 10 weeks, or 150g each week, in order to double his birth weight by 24 weeks.

87

⇝ One breast or two

This will largely depend on your cup size and how hungry your baby is. Most mums feed from both sides at each feed by weeks 10–12. Continue to offer baby both breasts freely and monitor poo colours. Yellow is good, green is bad. (See page 170.)

⇝ Feeding patterns

Many three-month-old babies still feed three-hourly during the day but have longer gaps at night. Continue feeding three-hourly during the day until baby is sleeping for 7–10 hours at night. If your baby suddenly changes his feeding pattern or your supply seems low, see page 158 for tips on how to boost your supply.

⇝ Overtiredness

To prevent overtiredness, have a clear end to the day that your baby expects and responds to. Introduce a bathtime and winding-down routine at a set time each day. By doing this you won't have sleep problems later on as your baby will be in a good routine (see page 114 for routines).

⇝ Bottle-feeds

Your baby should be fully able to breast- and bottle-feed well by now. If you haven't introduced a bottle-feed into your routine yet and want baby to be able to take a bottle when you go back to work, I would suggest that you get on to it as soon as possible. You can expect a great deal of resistance, so have a look at the practical tips on page 170.

⇝ Awake time

Your baby is able to be awake for 1 hour 45 minutes to 2 hours before becoming overtired. As his feeds are getting shorter, you now have more playtime between feeds.

Breastfeeding a four-month-old

Apart from the constant pulling off your breast to keep an eye on his surroundings, your baby is more relaxed about feeds by now. You may worry about whether he is getting enough, but when you try to feed him for longer, he quickly becomes very cross.

Take a step back and follow his lead. He may want to only feed for a short period in the morning but like to feed for a bit longer in the afternoon. Provided he is sleeping well at night, you can be confident that he is getting what he needs during the day.

↪ Feeding patterns and routines

Your feeds might still be three-hourly but may only last 10–15 minutes. This is perfectly normal. If you offer baby the breast at three hours and he only feeds for a few seconds, push your feed back by 30 minutes to offer him milk every three and a half hours instead. When he is a bit hungrier, he is likely to feed better. (See page 119.)

↪ Awake time

He should be doing a bit of tummy time every day now to help strengthen his back, open his lungs and give him a chance to explore how to use his hands, arms and legs. This is all preparation for crawling and moving about. Place toys and his favourite books around him, so that he has something to look at. When you lie him on a play mat, monitor his mood to ensure that he doesn't become over-stimulated. He'll usually be able to play for about 10 minutes before it all becomes too much. If he fixes his gaze away from his toys, cries or just looks like he is trying to get away, he has had enough.

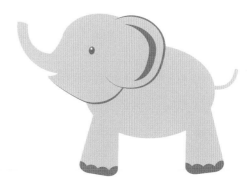

Breastfeeding a five-month-old

By five months your baby is an old hand at breastfeeding. Everything is easy. During feeds he gets what he needs before pulling off your breast. As he has places to go and people to see, he wants to get feeds over and done with as quickly as possible.

➡ Regular weight gain

Weight gain is only ever an issue if baby is gaining too little or too much weight. By five months monitor his weight gain loosely unless you are concerned about him. Focus on whether he reaches his developmental milestones instead.

➡ Feeding patterns and routines

Depending on how small or big your baby is, as well as your breast size, he can be feeding anywhere between two- and four-hourly during the day and three- and six-hourly at night. If your baby is still feeding every hour at night, get in touch with me or one of my team to sort this out, or see page 114 for suggestions on creating a routine.

➡ Bottle-feeds

If your baby is not taking a bottle by this point, you would probably be better moving straight on to a cup. There are many on the market but a soft spout is better as it is comfortable for him to feed from.

This stage is going to be messy, so I would suggest that you have two different-coloured cups; keep one in the kitchen for practising at meals and one in the bathroom, for practising at bathtime. He will soon get the hang of it and have fun trying until he gets it right.

➡ Awake time

He is better able to stay awake for close to two hours at a time now, so going to play groups, music or swimming classes becomes more manageable. He may have a longer sleep over lunchtime. Some babies prefer three short sleeps over the course of the day, others a longer sleep in the morning, over lunchtime or even in the late afternoon. As long as he is happy, don't worry about when he gets his daytime sleep.

Breastfeeding a six-month-old

By now your six-month-old is probably sitting up propped up by cushions and has good hand-to-mouth coordination. His pincer movements aren't well developed, so he can only grab big chunky things, but when he gets hold of them, he will hold on with a vice-like grip that's hard to break.

Your baby is getting ready for solids now, however, nutritionally milk trumps solids. Teething should have settled somewhat and you will have got used to baby pulling off mid-feed to flash your breast and nipples to all and sundry. Discreet public feeding, if you ever managed it, is long past and you probably don't even care about it anymore, which is great as breastfeeding your baby is natural.

➙ Feeding patterns and routines

If you haven't already introduced solids, you can start doing it now. Do it slowly so that you can continuously monitor baby's milk intake and sleeping patterns as you increase amounts of solids each week (see page 120).

➙ Awake time

At six months your baby will be happy to be awake for one and a half to two hours before becoming tired. If he needs to sleep sooner, let him, and if he isn't interested in having a nap at the two-hour mark but is happy, that is fine too. An active, busy baby may need more down time than a passive, relaxed little guy, so try not to compare your baby's sleep pattern to your friend's baby because they are different.

➙ Bedtime

Your days will have quite a nice pattern to them and baby should be settling easily for bedtime if you introduced a bathtime routine as well as a bottle-feed earlier on. The key with babies and children is consistency. The more consistent you are, the more settled your baby will be, as he knows what to expect.

91

Breastfeeding between months 6 and 12

Your baby may not be growing as quickly as he did in the first six months but in the second six months he is developing useful skills and becoming more independent. He will continue to refine his skills, learn to crawl, coast and walk in the next few months.

⇢ Regular weight gain

Your baby is on target to triple his birth weight by 12 months but there is really no need to worry about this, unless he is not gaining weight, is ill or poorly. If he is well, happy and healthy, you don't need to have him weighed at all and you can just get on with enjoying him.

⇢ Feeding patterns and routines

Feeding patterns are set by about six months so there aren't any dramatic changes to expect. Your baby will continue to feed three- to four-hourly during the day and have longer stretches of six to twelve hours at night. Feeds will be short but if your baby needs extra calories, he may decide to incorporate a longer feed at bedtime.

⇢ Bottle-feeds

You may decide now to introduce more bottle-feeds into your baby's day, perhaps in preparation for going back to work. Have a look at how to wean baby off the breast for tips on how to do this (see page 125).

Breastfeeding beyond the first year

Breastfeeding provides far more than just an immunity booster every time he feeds, it offers love, warmth and acceptance. It's actually quite handy to continue breastfeeding when your little one starts crawling, coasting or walking, because this is when he is most likely to come into contact with bugs and lurgies. As soon as he connects with your breast to feed, your body detects any new threats and produces anti-bodies to wipe them out. The immune-boosting properties in your milk is relative to volume, so your baby gets the same immunisation hit whether he is having a little or a lot of milk each day.

You'll know when to call time on breastfeeding as both you and baby will be ready to move on to new things. There is no rush or pressure to stop breastfeeding at 12 months. Many mums continue to feed beyond two years if that works for them.

Breastfeeding is a very emotive topic and stirs up a lot of feeling, which is why when it goes well, you feel like superwoman, but when it goes wrong, you feel absolutely miserable.

I have covered the complete breastfeeding journey over the last few chapters, with no bias or prejudice of where you start or end your journey. I want you to know that any breastfeeding you do, or any breast milk that your baby gets makes a difference. Even if you try and find that it doesn't work, you know that you gave it your best shot, and nobody can ask for any more from you.

CHAPTER 10

HOW TO BREASTFEED TWINS
YOU CAN DO IT

The idea of breastfeeding twins may seem daunting but once you get the hang of it, it can be relatively straightforward.

Your cup size, babies' age and size are the three most influential factors to determining how best to approach breastfeeding. Your priority should be to establish a good supply as quickly as possible as this enables you to breastfeed in the long term.

If you want to give breastfeeding twins a try, it is worth having some help either from your family and friends or a maternity nurse. They will be able to hold, wind or feed one baby while you take care of the other until everything settles down and you can manage both on your own. (See page 185 for Miskin Maternity details.)

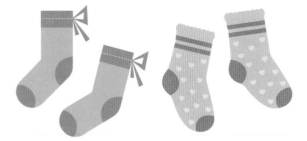

How to breastfeed twins

↣ Single feeding

It's easier to feed one baby at a time, waking the hungrier twin 30 minutes before feed time so that by the time baby number two wakes, baby number one has nearly finished his feed. You may need to use a dummy to placate the baby that is not being fed or pop him into a bouncy chair and jiggle him with your foot.

Once they are older, you can wake and feed both babies together to make time for yourself between feeds.

↣ Double feeding

Feeding both babies together is the quickest option but it only works well when your babies latch easily on their own. This is usually by 12 weeks. To ensure both babies feed from the more productive breast evenly, alternate which side they start on and then swap them over to the other side midway through each feed.

↣ Nipple shields

As nipple shields are firm, your twins have something firm to latch on to and you are able to latch each baby single-handedly. They also help keep your babies latched during the feed and the firm pressure on the babies' tongues keeps them awake and sucking.

↣ Breast compression

Use breast compression as much as possible to get milk into your babies at feeding times. This will help establish a good supply and ensure that your feeds are effective.

↣ Position for feeding twins

The underarm position is probably easiest if you are feeding your twins together, but if you are feeding one baby at a time you may prefer to use the cross-cradle position. (See page 44 and 46 for how to get both these positions right.)

Your babies will be happy with whatever you do, as long as they get their milk, cuddles and love. Often breastfeeding is easier one to one in the early days and double feeding is better when the babies are a bit older, more wakeful and focused.

You can use either the cross-cradle or underarm position in the early days when you are learning about your individual babies. Look at the positioning and latching chapters to learn how to line your baby up with your breast size.

TIP

Supply is driven by drainage not demand. The more you drain, the more you'll produce.

Feeding tips for small-sized breasts

Your cup size as well as your babies' size will indicate how best to approach breastfeeding.

➜ Small breasts plus small babies

The small-breast-and-baby combination is great as your babies will only need small amounts at each feed. Try feeding your babies together, using nipple shields if they struggle to latch. Ensure that you have a good feeding cushion so that they are high enough to reach the breast and get both cheeks touching the breast. (See page 42.)

The reason double feeding works for this combination is that your breasts are less likely to move once your babies have latched. As your babies are little and won't need much milk, your feeds will be over quickly. If you prefer to feed one baby at the time to start with that is absolutely fine too.

➜ Small breasts plus medium babies

As one baby is often hungrier than the other, try single feeding both babies at the start of the feed and then feed them together after their nappy change. This enables you to get as much as possible into each baby to start with so that they just need a lovely top-up to finish them off. It will speed up your feeds and help you to ensure that both babies are well fed by the end of the feed.

Remember to swap them over when they come back to the breast for a top-up feed. You can use nipple shields when you are ready to double feed to ensure that your babies latch easily.

➜ Small breasts plus hungry babies

You can try feeding one baby at a time but you'll probably find that combining breast- and bottle-feeds will be easier and more enjoyable for all of you. You have a few options, as follows:

• Breastfeed one baby and bottle-feed the other at each feed, alternating which baby breast- and bottle-feeds.
• Breastfeed both babies and finish off with a top up or bottle-feed.
• Express and split expressed milk between babies and allow them to suckle on your breast for comfort.

If you don't have enough milk to satisfy both babies, use formula to make up the difference and see page 158 for tips on how to boost your supply.

Any breast milk that your babies get is fantastic and some breast milk is better than nothing, so don't be put off combination feeding. If you find that breastfeeding, expressing and the like dominate your day and make you miserable, move on to bottle-feeds knowing that you have done your best.

Feeding tips for medium-sized breasts

↦ Medium breasts plus small babies

You will probably find feeding both babies together relatively easy, provided they are able to latch well, and you can use nipple shields if your babies struggle to latch. Once your babies are latched, tuck a rolled-up muslin behind their backs to keep them close to the breasts and free your hands. You can compress the breast to nudge them awake if you need to.

↦ Medium breasts plus medium babies

Try feeding both babies together for most of your feeds but consider doing at least one single feed with each baby during the day. When you single feed, express enough milk for one baby from both breasts and then feed the second baby from both breasts to ensure he gets enough milk too.

↦ Medium breasts plus hungry babies

You may find that one twin is hungrier – and this is very normal. You can decide whether you want to alternate breastfeeding and bottle-feeding or breastfeed both babies together and then just top up your hungrier baby with expressed milk or formula. (See page 104 for advice on when to express.)

Feeding tips for large-sized breasts

↦Large breasts plus small babies

You will have more than enough milk to feed your twins, but finding a comfortable position is often a common challenge for this combination. If it is easier, express and bottle-feed until your babies are bigger and able to latch comfortably without losing your breast easily.

↦Large breasts plus medium babies

This is really a great combination, as you will produce more than your babies need and they will be big enough to feed effectively but leave enough milk for you to express for bottle-feeds. Try feeding both babies together or you can alternate expressed feeds with breastfeeds to make life easier.

↦ Large breasts plus hungry babies

You'll have more than enough milk for your babies but as they are hungry, you may need to switch them over midway through the feed, so that both babies get to feed from your super-productive side. Use breast compression to keep the milk flowing and them happily feeding.

PART 3:
CREATING FLEXIBILITY

CHAPTER 11

HOW TO EXPRESS
WHAT YOU NEED TO KNOW

Your milk supply is driven and maintained by effective breast drainage, not demand, so it is worth knowing how to express should you find that your baby is not an efficient feeder to start with. By expressing you'll be able to establish and maintain a healthy supply until your little one is ready and able to take over and get milk directly from your breast. Whether you want to express occasionally or as a regular part of your day, there are so many effective pumps on the market to choose from that expressing is easy, simple and pain-free.

You may decide that, although breastfeeding is going well, you'd like somebody else to do a feed on occasion so that you are able to get some extra sleep, or you may like to know how to express milk for when you are away from your baby. We'll cover all the practical elements of expressing in this chapter.

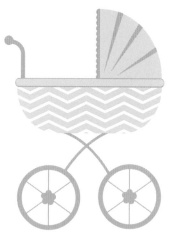

How to express

When you are trying to establish your supply, breastfeeding is not the best way to do this if your baby is too little, weak or young to drain your breasts effectively. In these situations you are better off expressing frequently to collect milk and create a healthy supply to start with. By establishing your supply first, you'll be better placed to return to breastfeeding later on.

Small breasts
• Express both breasts every two to three hours, day and night, to establish supply.
• Compress and massage your breasts to keep milk flowing.
• Power pump if your milk flow stops after 10 minutes. (See page 165).

Medium breasts
• Express both breasts every three hours.
• Compress your breast when milk flow slows or stops.
• Express for 20 minutes.

Large breasts
• Express both breasts every three to four hours.
• Compress your breast when milk flow slows or stops.
• Express until you get a little more than your babies need.
• This may only take 10–15 minutes.

EXPRESSING TIPS

If you are using a single pump, switch the pump between breasts when your milk stops flowing.

Only express what your baby needs, to avoid creating an oversupply problem, unless you intend to exclusively express, in which case you can express to drain both breasts.

If supply is low, express more frequently to boost your supply. Also see page 158 for tips on boosting low supply.

How to hand-express

Hand-expressing is the easiest way to collect droplets of colostrum that would just get lost in a pump funnel.

Before you express, place your hand on the breast and push your hand into it to flatten it against your ribcage. Hold for 10 seconds and then move your hand to another part of the breast, push into it and hold for 10 seconds. This is called breast compression and encourages a let-down.

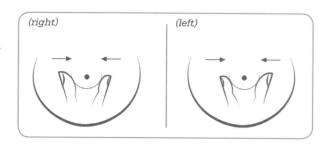

(right)   (left)

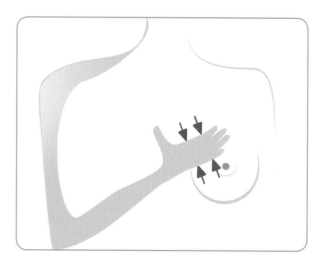

Once you have done this, work your way around the breast making small circular motions with your fingertips. If you are able to apply heat, such as a hot water bottle, wheat or cherry-stone bag, it will help move the colostrum down a little quicker.

Place your thumb at 3 o'clock and your middle and other fingers at 9 o'clock on the outer areola edge. You will feel that the breast tissue is lumpier or gritty here.

Gently bring your thumb and fingers together so that they almost touch through the breast tissue. Hold for 10 seconds and then release and pinch again. Work your way all round your areola.

You can either collect colostrum in a syringe or little cup. Once you have worked your way around the entire areola, you can move on to the second breast.

Move back and forth between breasts until you have enough milk or an hour has lapsed. Have a break and then repeat every three hours from start to start.

Once your milk is in and flowing effortlessly, you'll find using a breast pump easier. Your pump will come with instructions, so be sure to read through these and sterilise everything before baby arrives, so that you don't get caught on the hop.

How to choose the right pump

Different pumps suit different needs, so do some research and find one that meets all your criteria. The best pump to use is a hospital-grade double pump like the Medela Symphony, which you can hire from a local outlet. Google 'Medela Symphony pump rental' to find your nearest source. Get the 'pumping bra' from Amazon, so that both your hands are free to massage your breasts or hold an unsettled baby.

➜ Exclusive expressing
It's best to hire a hospital-grade double electric pump, preferably with the pumping bra to go with it.

➜ Regular expressing
Pumping both sides simultaneously is quicker and more effective but if you prefer to do one side at a time, a single pump is fine.

➜ Travel-friendly
If you travel a lot, opt for a pump that is easy to transport and use abroad.

You can start expressing regularly at around three weeks just before your baby's three-week growth spurt. If you are a second- or third-time mum, your milk will be in a lot sooner, so if you want to start expressing earlier, that is fine too.

As your milk supply is highest in the early morning (1am–4am) it is better to express at the start of the day. Express after the first two feeds of the day, usually 6am/7am and 9am/10am, to take advantage of your naturally high milk supply overnight.

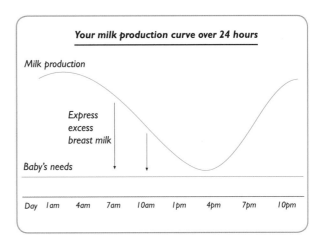

Your milk production curve over 24 hours

Milk production

Express excess breast milk

Baby's needs

Day 1am 4am 7am 10am 1pm 4pm 7pm 10pm

Your breast size will determine whether you express immediately after a feed or need to wait a bit. (See page 103.)

How to express effectively

- Ensure that your nipple is centred to the cylinder so that you don't get sore and so you can drain the entire breast evenly.
- Check that the cylinder comfortably fits around your nipple. If your nipples become sore or you see a white ring around the rim as your breast pulls into the cylinder, you need a bigger funnel.
- Keep the funnel in full contact with the breast to maintain suction, without pushing it into the breast too firmly. When the funnel indents the breast, you'll close milk ducts and prevent milk flow.
- Distract yourself so that you don't focus or stare at the pump. You'll let down more milk when you are relaxed about expressing rather than worrying about why it is not coming out.
- Keep the suction at a comfortable level and use breast compression to keep your milk flowing.
- Move back and forth between your breasts when you are compressing and no milk is coming through.
- Always express in place of a missed breastfeed to regulate breast drainage and prevent mastitis developing.

TIPS

Freeze milk in different volumes so that you can thaw what you need.

Never heat milk in the microwave as the heat is not evenly distributed and can burn baby's mouth and throat.

How to store, thaw and warm breast milk

Breast milk is a living fluid so it doesn't go off as quickly as formula, which is why storing guidelines are different and more flexible.

You can use one bottle per expressing session, even if you express from both sides at 7am. When you start your next expressing session at 10am, it is best to use a new or separate bottle. You can add breast milk to breast milk when the milk is the same temperature.

➻ Store breast milk
- At room temperature, out of direct sunlight for six hours.
- At the back of the fridge where it is coldest for five days.
- In the freezer compartment inside your fridge for two weeks.
- In the back of the freezer for three months.

➻ Thaw frozen breast milk
- Overnight in the fridge and use within 24 hours.
- At room temperature and use immediately.
- In a bowl of warm water and use immediately.

➻ Warm breast milk
Stand the bottle of milk in a bowl of hot water. Give it a shake and keep checking the temperature of the milk. Test it on your inner wrist, as this is most sensitive. It should feel neither hot nor cold when it is body temperature.

How to express according to your breast size

As your breast size determines storage capacity, it has a direct link to expressing, regardless of how much milk you produce over a day.

It's important to know that the pump doesn't drain the breast as effectively as your baby does. Don't worry if you only express small amounts, your baby is usually able to get 60ml more if he were to feed from the breast.

→ Small breasts (AA–D)

As you have restricted storage capacity, your challenge is to express enough for a feed without increasing your supply, as this compounds feeding challenges related to small breasts.

Volumes

You will probably find that baby drains the breast effectively, leaving very little to express. You may only be able to express 5–10ml at the end of a feed, but over time this quantity will increase.

Timings

Wait for 45 minutes to an hour after the feed before you express to allow your breasts to partly refill. If your baby feeds every two hours, you won't have time to express, so focus on feeding first. When he is bigger and has longer stretches between feeds, you can start expressing.

Breastfeeding after expressing

As your storage capacity is low, you need to allow as much time as possible between feeds to fill up. When you express, keep the session as short and effective as you can so that you have maximum refill time. Also see power pumping on page 165 for when you need to express a full feed quickly.

Top tips for effective expressing

- Express to accumulate milk and create a milk bank before introducing a bottle-feed. This helps you to get ahead without disturbing supply.
- Compress right from the start of the session. Use your fingertips to squeeze the breast so that you don't break the suction.
- Switch the pump, moving back and forth between both breasts, when your milk stops flowing.

Troubleshooting tips

- Get up early so that you can express an hour before your baby's first feed. This allows you express some milk and refill before baby's feed. You'll be able to get more milk this way. Pump for five minutes on each breast using compression to steal milk and have time to refill.
- Express between feeds throughout the day to accumulate expressed milk. This will enable you to express more milk at each sitting and leave time for your breasts to refill before baby's feeds.
- Use a double pump to reduce time spent expressing and to create more refilling time before your next feed.

⇸ Medium breasts (DD–G)

The amount you are able to express is largely dependent on how well your baby drains your breast. If your baby is little, expressing should be simple, but if he is very hungry, you may find yourself in the same position as a small-breasted mum.

Volume

As you have more glandular tissue and storage capacity you may be able to express 20–40ml immediately after the feed. This doesn't sound like much, but taking into account that you have fed your baby and the pump isn't as efficient as he is, it's a good start.

Timings

Expressing immediately after the feed is worth trying, especially if baby feeds less from one side. Even if he feeds evenly from both, you can try expressing immediately after as you have more storage capacity than a small-breasted mum.

Breastfeeding after expressing

Keep your expressing sessions effective to allow at least an hour between expressing and feeding. Expressing will be trickier when he goes through a growth spurt and feeds constantly. In which case, leave expressing until he is back to his three-hourly pattern.

Top tips for effective expressing

- Do a quick pump (5 minutes) on the side he fed from most and a longer pump (10 minutes) on the side he fed from least.
- If using a double pump, do 10 minutes on each with compression throughout.
- Try not to express more than what he needs in a full feed. (See page 111.)

Troubleshooting tips

- You'll have enough milk to feed baby if he wakes earlier than usual after expressing. Offer both sides and compress your breast throughout the feed. If he is still hungry, offer him the milk you expressed.
- Don't express during growth spurts. Instead feed him well so that he quickly falls back into his three-hourly feeding pattern and things get back to normal.

→ Large breasts (GG+)

Provided your breasts aren't great pretenders, expressing should be easy for you. However, you need to pay careful attention to the positioning of the funnel. As you have more breast tissue, you'll find it useful to massage the lower half of your breast while expressing to find any hidden blockages.

Volume

Depending on how hungry your baby is and whether he feeds from both sides, you'll be able to express 40–60ml at each expressing session. Be careful not to express more than he needs or your body will replace it and you'll develop an oversupply.

Timings

Express as soon after the feed as possible to drain what is naturally available. Don't delay expressing or your breasts will think it is an entirely new feed and ramp up your supply.

Breastfeeding after expressing

Keep your expressing sessions short and effective to create filling time before the next feed. You'll have more than enough milk in your breast after an express to feed baby if he wakes early.

Top tips for effective expressing

• Express from the side baby fed from and then the second side if you need more milk. If the second side feels full and achy, you can take the edge off that side to keep you comfortable until the next feed, even if you don't need the milk.
• Sit back so that the pump can comfortably tilt under the breast to prevent you losing suction or milk.
• Attach the pump to the breast when your breast is at rest. If you lift your breast, you will need to hold it in place throughout the entire session.
• Use breast compression to keep milk flowing while checking the breast for hidden lumps or knots.

Troubleshooting tips

• Lift your breast with a rolled-up muslin to get the pump into a better position.
• Only express what you need, instead of expressing to drain the breast, to prevent developing oversupply.
• If you don't get much milk, you may have less glandular tissue than expected. Express as if you are medium-breasted until your supply meets your baby's appetite.

When expressing hurts

When done correctly, expressing shouldn't hurt but if it does, you know that something is wrong. You will be able to tell from the state of your nipples what the most likely cause is. Here are a few common challenges you may encounter.

⇢ Purple nipples

When your suction is cranked up way too high, you'll break blood capillaries in your nipple, giving them a purple appearance. Turn the suction down so that it is at a comfortable level.

⇢ White nipples

White nipples are a result of blood flow being restricted to your nipple. Ensure that your pump funnel is the correct size and that your nipple is centred throughout the expressing session. Apply heat before and after expressing and turn down the suction.

⇢ Cracked, bleeding nipples

You can expect these with expressing if you have stubborn inverted nipples or if the pump funnel is too small and your nipple is squeezed into a small space. If your nipples are inverted, express with minimal suction and a lot of breast compression. Slowly work your way up to a stronger level of suction but be guided by your nipples.

How to express when you have thrush

You shouldn't freeze any milk you express while you are being treated for thrush. You can bottle-feed it to your baby while you are both being treated but if you freeze it, you will reintroduce thrush later on down the line.

If you have a lot of milk or even too much for baby, you will need to bin the excess milk so that there is no chance of re-infection later on. Sterilise all your expressing and bottle-feeding equipment, as well as any pacifiers too, as this is the best way of really getting rid of thrush completely.

Expressing is great if you want to create flexibility while providing all the milk your baby needs. Express according to your cup size and don't worry about volumes when you first start. If you only get small amounts, check that you are holding the pump correctly and know that the more you express, the more you will produce. Technique is important with everything, even bottle-feeding, as you will see in the next chapter.

CHAPTER 12

BREAST- AND BOTTLE-FEEDING
SIMPLE RULES TO FOLLOW

We live in a world where demands on our time are endless, and despite our best intentions, sometimes exclusive breastfeeding becomes unsustainable and bottles are introduced.

This chapter is about how you can combine breastfeeding and bottle-feeding, so that your little one enjoys the benefits of your milk for as long as possible.

Yes, there is a chance that by introducing bottle-feeds your supply may dip, but this is usually only the case if your supply is already low because your baby isn't draining your breast effectively, or you aren't told how to introduce formula while boosting or maintaining your supply.

I'm a great believer in a proactive, preventative and empowered approach to combined feeding. It can amount to more work than exclusive breastfeeding but if it works for you and your baby gets breast milk for an extended period, it's a good option to consider. ⸱

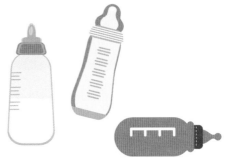

Good things to know about mixed feeding

To an adult, bottle-feeding seems simple and straightforward. For a baby who happily breastfeeds, bottle-feeding raises a number of challenges that many parents and nannies are oblivious to.

There is a concern that once you introduce a bottle-feed he will suddenly forget how to breastfeed or choose the easier option with a faster flow. Don't worry, this won't happen unless there is an underlying problem already. (See page 110 for common causes of refusing the breast after a bottle.)

The rules for combination feeding are simple:
• Establish a good milk supply by breastfeeding or expressing frequently in the first two weeks.
• Express in lieu of breastfeeds until you are ready to drop them altogether.
• Choose a lighter formula so it doesn't distort feeding patterns.
• Monitor baby's weight gain to ensure that you aren't overfeeding him.

Many mums want to express milk so that somebody else can do a feed while they get some rest. This is perfectly workable, provided you don't miss a feed entirely. If you are able to express enough milk for one full feed in the morning, express an hour before or after the feed you missed, so that your production is regular. (See routine for weeks 4–8 on page 118.)

↪ Breastfeeding and expressed milk combination

Where possible, express milk for bottle-feeds so that your body continues to produce 100 per cent of your baby's milk intake. (See page 99.)

↪ Breastfeeding and formula milk combination

When expressing doesn't work and you use formula at some feeds, ensure that when baby does breastfeed, he feeds well to maintain the supply you have available. The more milk you remove, the more your body replaces.

↪ Alternating breast- and bottle-feeds

This is a good option for when you go back to work. (See page 98.)

In short, you can mix and match breast- and bottle-feeds to fit in with your day, provided your breasts are emptied on a regular basis and you maintain your supply by removing only what your baby needs. As soon as you miss feeds altogether or drain your breasts in an ad hoc fashion, your supply will drop and you'll be vulnerable to developing mastitis.

Introducing a bottle-feed

Ideally, it is best to get breastfeeding established before you introduce bottles, sterilising, expressing and all that goes with it. If you introduce a bottle before breastfeeding is established, don't give up on breastfeeding. Many babies happily move between breast and bottle without any problem. In my practice, I often use bottle-feeds to teach babies to breastfeed.

Typically it takes a couple of weeks to get into a breastfeeding rhythm and to get your supply in line with baby's needs, so don't express before then unless you really need to.

You know that breastfeeding is established when your baby feeds well, is satisfied after feeds and gains weight nicely and your nipples are intact and your breasts feel comfortable.

It is important to stress here that not all babies can breastfeed effectively from birth, so if you have to express and bottle-feed your baby, do it without guilt. Persevere with expressing as regularly as you would breastfeed, to maintain your supply and get one-to-one help to get baby back on to the breast.

Why some babies prefer bottle-feeding

There are many valid reasons or circumstances when babies will prefer to bottle-feed rather than breastfeed, and these are just a few of them:
- Mums who don't produce enough milk and baby is hungry – it's simple survival.
- Mums who produce too much milk and baby finds the flow overwhelming.
- Babies who aren't able to breastfeed effectively or transfer milk. If their suck-to-swallow ratio is high, baby burns more calories than he banks because he is working so hard to get his milk.
- Babies who aren't able to hold on to, stabilise and suckle the breast without losing it due to birth compression or anatomical structures such as a tongue-tie or inverted nipples.
- Babies who have temporary post-birth cranial compression and can't breastfeed – it's simply mechanical.
- Babies who have a floppy larynx, trachea or epiglottis and can control milk flow better when bottle-feeding.

109

TIP

There's no expiry or cut-off date to get breastfeeding right. Keep your supply going so that there is plenty available for when your baby can feed properly.

NIPPLE/TEAT CONFUSION

True nipple/teat confusion, when a baby learns to feed from a bottle but forgets how to breastfeed, is not as rife as many of my clients are led to believe – having been told that if they give baby one bottle he will never again breastfeed.

What I find more frequently is what I call 'perceived nipple/teat confusion', where a totally reasonable and easily resolved problem causes temporary fussiness. Once it is resolved, baby will happily breastfeed without any problems.

This is not nipple/teat confusion, this is breastfeeding consultant confusion! We need to learn a lot more about how babies breastfeed and what happens during the feed when things aren't going well so that we can better support mum and baby when this happens.

↣ Choosing a bottle

Individual brands spend a lot of money marketing their products to make you feel like you are buying the best for your baby. The truth is that you won't know which bottle will suit your baby until he arrives and you can assess his palate.

Flat, wide-neck teats, which are currently in fashion, don't suit many baby's oral shape and this often leads to baby swallowing air. They may be suitable for baby when he is little and there isn't much space between his tongue and palate but are likely to cause problems as he gets older when the bottle doesn't fill his mouth properly.

I find the NUK standard neck teat, which is long and wide, the most compatible teat for a wide range of baby oral variations, including tongue-ties, as it often fills baby's mouth well, encouraging a lapping movement of the tongue.

TIP

If your baby can't breastfeed efficiently, he won't be able to feed easily from bottles such as the Medala Calma or Habermann baby bottles, which mimic breastfeeding.

How much to offer your baby

It is important to ensure that your baby gets enough milk at each feed but doesn't consistently overfeed. When your baby gets used to having a lot more milk than he needs from a bottle it makes it harder for your supply to catch up.

This changes rapidly and varies from baby to baby, but the important measurements to know are as follows.

➡ First week

Your baby's tummy is only the size of a Malteser on day 0 but quickly grows and increases to the size of a ping-pong ball by day 7. For the first week, calculate volume per feed as follows:

Baby's age in days x 10ml per feed.
So:
1 day old x 10ml = 10ml per feed.
2 days old x 10ml = 20ml per feed.

Offer feeds every three to four hours, calculating from the start of one feed to the start of the next. Feed baby earlier if he is hungry.

➡ Second to twelfth week

Calculate your baby's feeds according to his weight. Round up to the nearest ½kg or lb to ensure that you offer him a bit more than he needs. You know that he has had enough if he is full and has left a little milk in the bottle.

➡ Metric calculation

Baby's weight in kg x 180ml, then divide by the number of feeds in 24 hours.

E.g. 4kg x 180ml, divide by 8 feeds in 24 hours.
720ml divided by 8 = 90ml per feed every 3 hours.

➡ Imperial calculation

Baby's weight in lbs x 3oz, divide by the number of feeds in 24 hours.

E.g. 8lbs x 3oz, divide by 8 feeds.
24oz divided by 8 = 3oz per feed every 3 hours
This is a generous calculation as baby only needs 2.5oz/lb, but 3oz is easier to calculate.

How to hold your baby

In order to control milk flow, sit your baby upright, either leaning against your body or facing you. Support his upper back and head with one hand and hold the bottle with the other.

Keep the bottle horizontal so that baby draws the milk through at a neutral gravitational pull. (*Fig. 1*)

As the bottle empties, lean baby back but keep the bottle mostly horizontal. (*Fig. 2*)

Don't lie baby back and tip the bottle down into his mouth until the bottle is nearly empty. Gravity will encourage a faster flow and your baby won't be able to breathe because the milk will just pour into his mouth if you do this at the start of the feed.

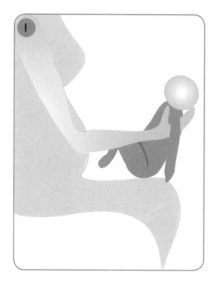

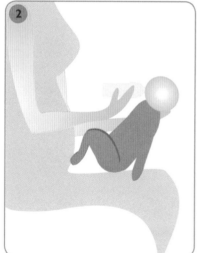

112

TIP

The teat doesn't have to be full of milk, only the tip of the teat or the exit point should be covered with milk, to avoid baby sucking in air. You will hear when this has changed.

Getting baby to take a bottle-feed

You can encourage baby to bottle-feed by mimicking breastfeeding with the bottle. Using the tip of the teat, tap baby's upper lip a couple of times then place the teat on baby's upper lip and wait for him to tip his head back and latch. If baby is sleepy or little, you can tap the corners of his mouth, teasing him a little until he roots and looks for the bottle.

Resist the temptation to push the bottle into baby's mouth, as this will dull his rooting reflex, which is important for effective latching on to your breast.

↦ Paced feeding

You can control how quickly your baby drinks his milk by monitoring how often he pauses to catch his breath. If he doesn't do this after every 5–10 swallows, take the bottle away from him and allow him to catch his breath.

By pacing his feeds, you can reduce wind intake and prevent unsettled or fussy behaviour after the feed has finished.

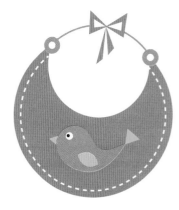

There is a lot of guilt and pressure to breastfeed exclusively without ever introducing artificial teats. I'm of the mindset that you need to do what works for you and your baby so that he thrives and you love being a mum. You may find that for some reason you need to offer bottles regularly, and you may even use formula when you have low supply to give yourself a chance to refill and ensure that your baby gets some breast milk for a longer period. You may even decide to introduce a regular bottle-feed to create a bit of structure. We'll look at routines in the next chapter.

CHAPTER 13

HOW TO SET A ROUTINE
TO GIVE YOUR DAY MORE STRUCTURE

You shouldn't feel any pressure to get your baby into a routine but if you naturally like routine and want to have an idea of what to expect and when, you can loosely follow the timings set out below. They will never be this neat, so don't fret if your day looks very different.

To ensure that you always have enough milk, feed according to your cup size and your baby's needs. Most mum-and-baby combinations feed roughly three-hourly by week 5, but if your baby still feeds two-hourly during the day in order to sleep longer at night, that is fine too.

There is no need to start your day at a set time; instead, leave your baby to wake naturally in the morning and calculate your next feed accordingly, if this suits you better.

Before we look at routines, here are five simple ways to help you decide whether baby needs to feed, burp or sleep.

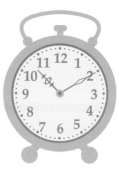

The hour-and-a-half rule

In order to settle easily, baby's stomach should be full and he shouldn't be overtired or stimulated. There is a small window of opportunity and this rule will help you get it right.

The hour-and-a-half rule in theory is:

1. Your baby's stomach will be empty one and a half hours from the start of the feed.

2. He will start to feel overtired and will struggle to settle on his own one and a half hours from when he wakes.

3. A baby will not go to sleep on an empty tummy but will sleep through an empty tummy.

The hour-and-a-half rule in practice is:

Last fed:

 less than one and a half hours ago but not settling:
   • may have wind that needs to come out.
   • may be tired and want to sleep.
 more than one and a half hours ago and not settling:
   • may be tired but, as his tummy is empty, you need to feed first before you settle him.

Last woke:

 less than one and a half hours ago:
   • shouldn't be overtired unless he has had too much stimulation.
   • may be hungry or have trapped wind.
 more than one and a half hours ago:
   • most probably tired and wants to sleep.
   • feed again if your last feed started more than one and a half hours ago, then put him to bed quickly.

Some babies seem tired and ready for bed sooner than one and a half hours, while others seem happy to stay awake for longer. Where possible, it's best to get baby to feed well and efficiently at feeding times. If feeds go on for ages, your feeds will merge together and you'll be pinned to the sofa for hours.

The one-hour rule

Always allow baby to sleep for at least an hour before you wake him up for a feed. This may mean that you push back the start of a feed a little bit in order to accommodate this, but it is well worth doing.

If baby is not well rested he won't feed effectively and this often leads to snack feeds, interrupted sleep patterns and overtiredness.

115

TIP

If you aren't coping with the frequency of your baby's feeds, get in touch with me or one of my team (see page 185).

Little finger test

When you offer your baby a clean little finger to suck, he will do one of three things:
- He will suck frantically = hungry
- He will suck and become sleepy = tired
- He won't suck or become fractious = needs to burp

This is a quick and easy test for you to use, in combination with the two rules above, to decide whether or not to feed or wind baby before putting him down for a sleep.

As babies don't always just go to sleep as soon as you put them down, it is good to know these two additional tips too.

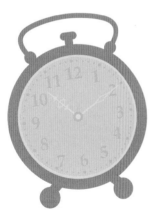

Cycle of 'littles'

When your baby only does a little feed, his stomach empties before one and a half hours and then won't go to sleep as his stomach is empty sooner. If you are stuck in a cycle of little feeds and little sleeps, you need to make a plan to get as much milk into baby at your next feed and encourage longer gaps between feeds.

If you are small-breasted, you will find that your breasts just don't have time to refill enough to give baby a full feed and knock him out. As he doesn't have a Christmas lunch feeling of fullness, he doesn't go into a deep sleep. Offer him a top up of expressed milk or formula after your feed, to fill him up properly, so that he goes to sleep and gives you more time to fill up before the next feed.

If you are medium- to large-breasted, ensure that you are doing a two-part feed and waking baby up mid-feed, in order to get as much milk into him, so that he settles for longer between feeds. This will be better for baby as he'll be better rested and prevent you developing an oversupply.

'Crying up' or 'crying down'

Once your baby is in his crib, it can be hard to know whether to give him space to settle or nip back in if he is crying. The trick is to listen to his cries. If they are escalating (crying up) go in quickly and calm him down before resettling. If his cries are slowing down, have slight pauses or breaks in between (crying down), give him space to settle himself.

Routine suggestions

Here are some routines that you can use. Feel free to change the timings to suit your baby if he prefers to wake at 8am or is an early riser and starts his day at 6am. The reason I like to start your day around 7am, is that it is not too early or too late and it enables you to get as many feeds into baby during the day as possible. This all leads to more sleep at night.

↪ Basic routine – weeks 0–2
Breastfeed three-hourly start to start, day and night, until your baby regains his birth weight.

Feeding times		Expressing times
7am	7pm	None
10am	10pm	
1pm	1am	
4pm	4am	

↪ Basic routine – week 2
Once your baby has regained his birth weight, leave him to wake for feeds after your last feed at night.

Feeding times		Expressing times
7am	7pm	None
10am	10pm	
1pm	Baby led	
4pm	Baby led	

↪ Basic routine – week 3
Create a bathtime and bedtime routine to mark the end of your day. By offering a split feed at 6pm, you get more of his daily calories into him before the night, so it encourages better sleep for the whole family.

Offer baby a small feed or one breast at 6pm while you run his bath. Then bath, dry and dress him and offer him a big long feed in his darkened nursery before putting him down for the night. Let him wake for feeds after his 10pm feed.

Feeding times		Expressing times
7am	6pm, bath, 7pm	None
10am	10pm	
1pm	Baby led	
4pm	Baby led	

117

TIP

If you want to breastfeed for six months, don't drop any feeds before week 14 or your supply will dwindle.

➜ Basic routine – weeks 4–8

Introduce a late-night bottle-feed between weeks 3 and 5 if you want baby to be able to do both. You will need to express after the 7am and 10am feeds to get enough milk for his bottle-feed. You also need to express at 9pm in lieu of the 10pm feed, to maintain your supply. You can freeze the milk you express at night to create a milk bank for later on. (See page 98 for expressing tips.)

Feeding times	Expressing times
7am	8am
10am	11am
1pm	9pm
4pm	
6pm, bath, 7pm	
10pm (bottle)	
Baby led	
Baby led	

Some babies don't like being woken for a 10pm bottle-feed; instead they prefer to have a breastfeed before their bath and a bottle-feed at 7pm, then sleep through to 2am. Try both options and see what works best for your baby. (*Fig.1*)

➜ Basic routine – weeks 8–12

If you want to encourage baby to have a longer lunchtime sleep, you can just tweak your feeding times like this:

Feeding times	Expressing times
7am	8am
10am	9pm
12.30pm	
3pm	
6pm, bath, 7pm	
10pm (bottle)	
Baby led	
Baby led	

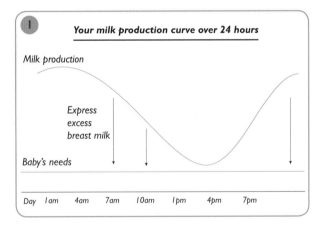

Your milk production curve over 24 hours

Milk production

Express excess breast milk

Baby's needs

Day 1am   4am   7am   10am   1pm   4pm   7pm

↦ Basic routine – weeks 12–16

At some point your baby won't feed well on a three-hourly feeding pattern anymore, so you can begin to increase the gaps between feeds.

Feeding times	Expressing times
7am	8am
10.30am	11.30am (optional)
2pm	9pm (optional)
3pm	
7pm	
10pm (bottle)	
Baby led	
Baby led	

- Express both breasts after the 7am and 10.30am feeds. If you want to drop the 9pm express, just express a little less each night until there is no milk.
- If you aren't able to express much at 11.30am, drop this session but keep your 9pm expressing session going to maintain supply. Offer him a formula bottle-feed at 10pm.
- If your baby wakes earlier than 10pm, offer him a top up with the milk you expressed the night before, after his bath, rather than another breastfeed.

↦ Basic routine – weeks 16–24

Your baby will prefer to feed four-hourly at some point between four and six months. This creates space in your day to introduce solids (see page 120). This is what your timings will now look like:

Feeding times	Expressing times
7am	8am (optional)
11am	9pm (optional)
3pm	
7pm	
10pm (bottle)	
Baby led	
Baby led	

You can drop your late-night express if you are offering your baby a bottle of formula at 10pm and your supply is buoyant during the day.

Your baby gets most of his nutrients from milk for the first year, so there is no rush or pressure to introduce solids. As you get ready to take a step back and supplement your milk feeds with solid foods, it's good to know how to do it so that your baby gets the right balance of milk and solids to thrive.

CHAPTER 14

HOW TO INTRODUCE SOLIDS
MOVE FORWARD WITHOUT REGRESSING

At some point between four and six months, you'll start introducing solid meals into your baby's day. There is absolutely no rush to start solids if your baby is full and content on his milk feeds. Some babies seem hungrier and ready for solids sooner than other babies, so follow your baby's lead and don't feel pressured to start earlier than you think is necessary.

It's normal to feel apprehensive about a new development or milestone, and introducing solids certainly gets your heart racing. To start with you'll watch baby like a hawk, ready to apply all skills learnt at your baby first-aid course. The first feeds are usually uneventful and meal times become easy and relaxed as you learn to trust your baby's ability to gum, spit out or swallow food he deems acceptable.

If there are allergies in the family, it is best to delay introducing solids or if you feel that your baby is just too hungry to go without them, get advice from a dietician to ensure that you introduce suitable foods.

In this chapter, we'll address the practicalities of introducing solids.

Know when your baby is ready for solids

Before introducing solids your baby needs to be able to sit up on his own, hold his head up and have good hand-to-mouth skills.

To start with, your baby will only be able to pick up large chunky objects, such as a roast potato, but as he grows he will find it easier to pick up smaller objects.

Theoretically, your baby will only be able to pick up and eat vegetables or foods that are safe (in size) and this is why baby-led weaning is such a popular option. (See more about this on the website, www.babyledweaning.com.)

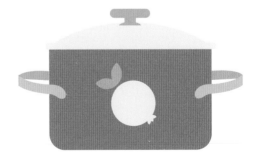

How to introduce solids

Before the age of 12 months, milk is more nutritionally valuable than solids, so don't be in a rush to introduce solids. Your baby needs a certain number of calories each day and when you start introducing solids the first foods will include puréed apple, pear and carrot, which are all low in calories.

Prioritising your baby's calorie intake is the easiest way to approach introducing solids. If you can see that he is filling up on puréed apple instead of creamy milk, you need to make the necessary changes to prevent this.

➥ Introduce feeds in line with baby's size
Your baby's size will give you a good idea of how to approach solids without affecting your milk supply.

Small babies
Only offer one meal a day for five to seven days while you monitor changes in feeding, sleep or pooing patterns. If there are no changes, add another solid meal (1 teaspoon of baby rice + 15ml of breast milk or formula). Then another meal is added a few days later. This works well for small babies as they will have a small stomach capacity and milk intake is easily displaced.

Days 1–5	1 small meal a day
Days 6–11	2 small meals a day
Days 12–18	3 small meals a day

Big babies

Big babies will feel frustrated by small portions, so instead of doing three small meals you can gradually add an additional teaspoon of food to your baby's first solid meal. Keep monitoring your baby's feeding, sleep and pooing patterns and if nothing changes move to introduce the second meal of the day. Don't increase the amount of baby rice too quickly or your baby will become constipated.

Days 1–5	1 small meal a day (1 teaspoon baby rice + 15ml breast milk)
Days 6–11	1 medium meal a day (1 teaspoon baby rice + milk + 1 teaspoon puréed apple)
Days 12–18	1 large meal a day (1 teaspoon baby rice + milk + 2 teaspoons puréed apple)

➡ Introduce one new food at a time

Always introduce one new food at a time and use the same food for three days before adding another. This way you can keep track of which foods your baby likes and any negative reactions your baby has to individual foods.

➡ Offer new foods in the morning or early afternoon

It is better to give baby solids at the start of the day so that you can watch him for any reactions and if you need to dash to the doctor, everything is open and accessible.

➡ Vary the foods you give him

As soon as you have introduced three solid meals and find that he is still sleeping well at night, you can introduce new flavours. Keep the portion sizes the same while you try him out on different foods.

➡ Offer solids as close to the end of a breastfeed as possible

This will ensure that he has as much time as possible for his tummy to empty before his next breastfeed is due. By doing it this way, you will protect your supply and ensure that he gets his milk feed first, which is more important than solids.

When to introduce solids into your day

Always offer your breast first, then he can take as much milk as he needs and the solids he has will complement breastfeeding rather than overshadow it.

Your day will now look something like this:

7am	Breastfeed
8am	Offer small portion of solids
11am	Breastfeed
3pm	Breastfeed
7pm	Breastfeed

Do this for two to three days then introduce a second solid feed into your day.

7am	Breastfeed
8am	Offer small portion of solids
11am	Breastfeed
12pm	Offer small portion of solids
3pm	Breastfeed
7pm	Breastfeed

Again, do this for a day or two, keeping an eye on your baby's feeding patterns. If baby suddenly breastfeeds more or you feel that your supply is dropping, you could be introducing solids too quickly.

The last feed in which you introduce solids is at teatime. If you feel that he is ready to have a third portion of solids, without this affecting his bedtime feed, you can introduce the third solid feed into your day.

7am	Breastfeed
8am	Offer small portion of solids (1–3 teaspoons)
11am	Breastfeed
12pm	Offer small portion of solids (1–3 teaspoons)
3pm	Breastfeed
4pm	Offer small portion of solids (1–3 teaspoons)
7pm	Breastfeed

➜ Solids and baby's lunchtime nap routine

This routine is usually good for babies who are roughly eight to nine months old.

7am	Breastfeed (big feed)
8am	Offer portion of solids (1–3 tablespoons)
10.30am	Snack (puréed fruit and rice cake)
12pm	Offer portion of solids (1–3 tablespoons)
12.30pm	Breastfeed (big/small feed)
1–3pm	Sleep
3pm	Breastfeed (big/small feed)
5pm	Offer portion of solids (1–3 tablespoons)
7pm	Breastfeed (big feed)

Your baby will start to have less breast milk at lunchtime and more solids. This is ok, as he will have a bigger feed when he wakes from his sleep. Some babies prefer to have a bigger feed after their solids and then a small feed when they wake up.

You will see that your baby has a big feed first thing in the morning and a big feed before bed. He will have another big feed either before or after his lunchtime nap, depending on which he prefers.

Can you see that your baby is now getting ready to drop either the 12.30pm or 3pm feed? This will leave you with the 7am, a lunchtime feed and a 7pm feed.

As your baby's solid portion sizes increase he will drop the lunchtime feed by 11 months.

➜ Introducing snacks as well as meals

The solid portion sizes will be a lot bigger and will comprise of two helpings: one savoury and one sweet.

Your baby will also have a mid-morning snack and a mid-afternoon snack. This is useful when you are out and about with baby, just to keep him going.

Some babies love having a breastfeed before their big lunchtime nap. If your baby is keen on breastfeeding here, go with it; soon he will be independent and disinterested.

7am	Breastfeed
8am	Breakfast (usually porridge and a fruit pot)
10.30am	Snack and drink
12.30pm	Lunch and pudding
1–3pm	Sleep
3pm	Fruit and drink
5pm	Solids
7pm	Breastfeed or bottle then bed

When you are ready, you can swap the 7pm breastfeed for a bottle-feed. The last feed you will drop is the 7am feed, as this is when your milk supply is highest.

Introducing solids is fun and marks a new chapter in your baby's life, but don't feel pressured to introduce solids before you feel that baby is ready. Focus on feeding according to your anatomy so that your supply is abundant and meets his needs.

CHAPTER 15

HOW TO WEAN YOUR BABY OFF THE BREAST
MAKE THE TRANSITION GENTLE

Once you have decided to wean your baby off your breast, you need to know how to do it safely and what your options are. I like to mention this as many mums think that once they start dropping breastfeeds, they have to drop all breastfeeds. The truth is that you can drop feeds that aren't suitable to your day and keep the ones that are. Many mums find that keeping one or two feeds a day works really well.

When it comes to weaning your baby off your breast, it is vital that you know how to do it without running into unexpected and unnecessary problems. The trick is to do it really slowly while keeping your breasts relatively well drained to avoid blockages and mastitis developing.

If for some reason your breasts become inflamed, you'll find all the tips you need in the engorgement chapter to resolve challenges and get back on track.

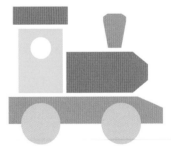

How to drop feeds before week 3

I want to start here, as many mums want to know how to drop feeds safely when they find that breastfeeding doesn't work. If you have made the difficult decision to stop breastfeeding so soon, the last thing I want is for you to develop mastitis on your way out.

When dropping feeds this early into breastfeeding, you can easily develop breast congestion and pain. You really have to be careful and vigilant for any congestion as your milk supply is very high and your hormones are all over the place. If you develop any congestion, have a quick look at the next chapter for essential tips for managing engorgement (see page 131).

Before you start dropping feeds, think about how you are going to replace them. You can either give baby a bottle of expressed milk from the previous day, your milk bank or from your early-morning expressing sessions (see page 98 for expressing tips) or you can give baby formula.

This is the order of how to drop your feeds in line with your supply.

10pm feed

You can either substitute this feed with the breast milk you expressed after the first and second feed, or you could offer formula at this stage. Express both breasts at 9pm in lieu of the feed to prevent mastitis. Gradually express less until you don't need to express at all.

4pm feed

Your supply is naturally low at this point, so it makes sense to take advantage of that and continue feeding when your supply is naturally high. You also space drainage by dropping alternate feeds.

10am feed

This evens out the feeds so that you develop a pattern where you keep one feed and drop one, so that you do not feel overly full or overly empty during the day.

4am feed

Continuing with the 'keep one, drop one' approach, you can now drop the 4am feed.

As your milk supply is naturally high at 4am, you may feel like you need to express a bit of milk in order to last until the morning. Only express to take the edge off; you don't want to over-express here, or you may become dependent on expressing and that really defeats the whole object of dropping feeds.

If bottle-feeding, be careful not to offer baby too much milk here or he will not be hungry to feed again at 7am and will throw your feeding pattern right out of the window.

1pm feed

As your milk supply is lowest between 1pm and 4pm, the next feed to drop is the 1pm feed, which leaves you with 7am, 7pm and 1am. Your milk supply is still pretty high at 1am so it is better to drop the 1pm first.

1am feed

Once you have dropped this feed, you will be left with 7am and 7pm.

The seventh and eighth feeds to drop

You will now be at a point when you only have the 7am feed and the 7pm feed after baby's bath. Most mums keep these two feeds going for as long as possible, even if or when baby is on formula feeds during the day.

If you are not home and your baby is desperate for a feed before his bath, his carer can give him a small bottle of expressed milk before his bath and you can feed him afterwards.

It is quite possible that your baby's feeding pattern has a life of its own, so just write down the times at which your baby regularly feeds and apply the principles above. It's not as daunting as it seems once you get started. Also have a look at the oversupply chapter (page 166) for tips on how to reduce your supply safely.

↱ Dropping feeds for older babies

Here are some timelines to show you in which order to drop feeds when your baby is older. The same principles apply in that you:

• Start by dropping the 10pm first, then drop your lowest of the remaining feeds.
• Aim to drop one, keep one feed to space feeds evenly throughout the day.
• Ensure that your breasts are drained evenly to avoid blockages.
• Always leave the 7am feed to last as this is when your supply is highest and dropping this feed early often leads to mastitis.
• Give yourself at least one week to drop each feed, so that you don't rush it.

If your baby feeds every three and a half hours, starting at 7am, and sleeps through the night, this is what your timeline looks like:

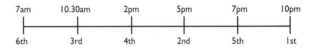

If your baby feeds every four hours, starting at 7am, and sleeps through the night, this is what your timeline looks like:

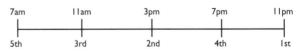

How to drop feeds without developing mastitis

Drop one feed at a time and only drop one feed a week. Drop feeds as slowly as possible, to allow your body and your baby to become accustomed to the changes. By giving yourself time, your hormones will remain stable and you will be able to manage breast lumps or engorgement effectively.

Some mums find that they have milk in their breasts for weeks, months or even years after they have dropped their final feed. This is normal and there is no need to express or fret about it.

TIPS TO DROP FEEDS SAFELY

The first feed you drop
is the 10pm feed.

You need to spread your feeds
evenly throughout the day, so aim
to keep one, drop one

The last feed you drop completely
is the 7am feed.

➜ Here are two easy options to reduce your supply:

Breastfeed and top up

This is the gentlest way to wean baby off the breast and definitely my preferred method.

Starting with the feed when your supply is lowest, you offer baby a breastfeed but reduce the length of the feed by five minutes and then top baby up with formula. As your supply is low, you are less likely to become engorged when you shorten feeding times.

Continue to shorten your chosen feed and increase the top up until baby is only on a bottle-feed. Once you have dropped the feed completely and your breasts feel comfortable, you can move on to the next feed you want to drop.

Bottle-feed and express

You will know that this is the best method if your baby is hungry, insatiable at each feed and you are very sore. You will offer baby a full bottle-feed at the feed you wish to drop. Once baby is settled, you can express to take the edge off your breast. Depending on how much milk you produce, this may be 60–90ml. You can then offer this milk for baby's bottle-feeds.

Gradually reduce the amount of milk you express at your chosen feed until you no longer have to express. When your breast feels comfortable, you can move on to the next feed you want to drop.

How to introduce formula

Formula is heavier than breast milk and, as it is different to what your baby expects, it's great if you can make the transition easier.

➜ Before you introduce formula

Formula has evolved, so it is good to speak to your GP about which formula would be most suitable for your baby. It is even more important if there is a history of allergies and skin sensitivities in the family.

At first you will be offering a combination of breast milk and formula, and as breast milk is so light and so readily absorbed by your baby's body, it is best to use a light formula rather than one that is heavy and filling. Don't use formulas 'for hungry babies' when you first introduce it, as these are quite heavy and will distort your baby's feeding pattern.

When you are ready to formula-feed, introduce the formula gradually so that you can tell whether baby is comfortable with the one you have chosen. If his poos turn slimy green or he starts throwing up, he is not getting on with the one you have introduced, so go back to your GP.

➜ Combine breast milk and formula to start with

Where possible, offer your baby a mixture of breast milk and formula.

• Start with three parts breast milk to one part formula. (E.g. 120ml feed = 90ml breast milk/30ml formula.) Do this for a couple of days and then increase the amount of formula and decrease the amount of breast milk.

• Move to two parts breast milk to two parts formula. (E.g. 120ml feed = 60ml breast milk/60ml formula.) Do this for a couple of days and then increase the amount of formula again.

• Move to one part breast milk and three parts formula. (E.g. 120ml = 30ml breast milk/90ml formula.)

➜ Irregular feeding patterns

If your feeds are all over the place and you choose to drop the late-night feed first, pick a time that this feed usually falls at, say 10pm. Regardless of how chaotic your feeds are during the day, at 10pm you apply your milk-dropping strategies until you have successfully dropped that feed. Do the same for all your feeds until you have successfully dropped them.

➜ Frequent night feeds

I would encourage you to still follow the feeding model timings. Once your baby moves on to a full bottle-feed at 10pm and then again at 4pm, he will be getting more of his daily calories at those feeds, so he should start to sleep longer for you at night and your daytime feeds will become more predictable and regular.

The most important thing to take away from this chapter is to make the transition slowly. If you become engorged or develop breast congestion, you know that you are moving too quickly.

PART 4:
TROUBLESHOOTING

CHAPTER 16

HOW TO MANAGE ENGORGEMENT
ESSENTIAL KNOW-HOW FOR A SPEEDY RECOVERY

When your milk 'comes in' and your breasts are hot, heavy and achy, we say that you are engorged. Even though you are sore and feel very uncomfortable, engorgement is normal and is not mastitis. Your breasts will settle down in a couple of days, once they get a measure of how much milk your baby needs.

All the information you find in this chapter can be applied at any stage of breastfeeding as soon as your breasts become hot, firm and swollen (also see my tips on page 142). If you find that a particular part of your breast seems to become repeatedly inflamed and sore, see Chapter 18 for more insight.

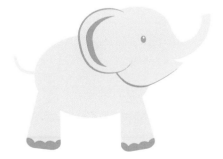

Managing engorgement

Engorgement is different for every mum. Sometimes it comes on suddenly, other times gradually. Some mums find that they don't become engorged at all. Often this is a reflection of your breast size and storage capacity.

Essentially you have two challenges to resolve. Firstly, you want to ensure that your baby can latch effectively, without creating nipple damage and pain. Secondly, you want to ensure that your baby is able to drain your breast well both to reduce swelling and inflammation and to secure a healthy milk supply. If your baby latches and feeds well, your supply will settle down but still meet your baby's needs. (*Fig. 1*)

Your body uses breast fullness after feeds to measure how much milk to produce and will only replace the milk that baby drains. Your supply will gradually decrease until it is in line with what your baby needs. (See page 21.)

↪ How to facilitate a good latch

As the majority of your glandular tissue is found just behind your nipple and areola (see page 18), this area will be full and very firm when your breast is engorged. This makes latching harder for your baby, as he isn't able to scoop up areola. In this situation you need to soften your areola, so that your breast is soft and pliable for baby to latch.

• Place your index and middle fingers together on either side of your nipple. Use your fingertips to gently push the milk collected here back into the breast. (*Fig. 2*.) Push in and hold for five seconds, then do top and bottom. (*Fig. 3*.)

• Work your way around your entire nipple until your areola is soft enough for baby to latch.

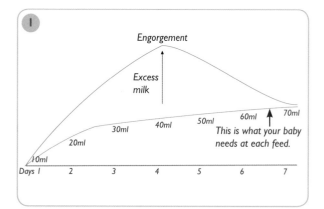

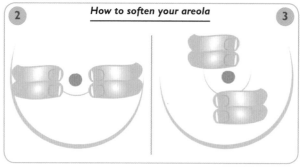

1 Engorgement

Excess milk

10ml · 20ml · 30ml · 40ml · 50ml · 60ml · 70ml

This is what your baby needs at each feed.

Days 1 · 2 · 3 · 4 · 5 · 6 · 7

2 3 *How to soften your areola*

How to calm your breast for better milk drainage

Normally, your milk ducts are naturally collapsed and only dilate to allow milk through. When your breast is inflamed and swollen, there isn't room for your ducts to dilate and this can lead to poor milk flow and drainage. To rectify this, here are a few simple steps you can follow before breastfeeding.

1. Apply something from the freezer to your breasts for 10–15 minutes to cool them and reduce swelling. This creates room for your ducts to open and let the milk out.

2. Apply a hot, wet facecloth to your nipple and areola. Using your fingertips, gently push the milk just behind the areola back into the breast, through your facecloth. Refresh your cloth and repeat until your areola is nice and soft.

3. Latch baby using the Pinch and Pop technique (see page 54) and feed according to your breast size (page 79).

4. Use breast compression to drain your breast effectively.

5. Apply something from the freezer to your breasts at the end of the feed.

> ### TIP
> If your breasts are hard but not hot, you probably have a lot of retained IV fluid.

How to manage engorgement according to your breast size

Your breast size influences how tight and uncomfortable you feel when you first become engorged. Here are some tips on how to manage engorgement based on your breast size.

⇢ Small breasts

Feed from both breasts every three hours. If your baby only feeds for 10 minutes, do 5 minutes on each. Massage the breast, particularly the upper bit close to your armpit, to ensure good drainage. Bring your feeds closer together if baby is willing, for more relief. Once your breasts feel better, feed according to your breast size (see page 79).

⇢ Medium breasts

Feed from both sides every three hours, swapping breasts after five minutes. Move back and forth between them until baby is full so that he drains them evenly. If one side flares up, focus on only feeding from one side per feed and expressing just enough off the other side to take the edge off your fullness. Once your breasts feel better, feed according to your breast size (see page 80).

⇢ Large breasts

Feed from one side per feed every three hours, alternating which side you start on. Express the tiniest amount of milk off the second side if you need to, to feel comfortable. Once your breasts feel better, feed according to your breast size (see page 81).

How and when to express when engorged

Your breasts are trying to gauge how much milk your baby needs, so you'll confuse them if you start expressing too early. The more you drain from the breast, the more you will produce, so try not to express if possible until your supply has settled.

However, if your baby is not feeding and you feel like you are going to pop, do one complete express of both breasts to wipe the slate clean. Thereafter, only breastfeed so that your body gets a measure of how much to produce.

↪ Too much IV fluid
If you were given a lot of IV fluid during labour, you'll find that your breasts remain 'full' for longer. Your breasts will be hard but cool instead of hot. You may notice that your baby does clear wees instead of the dark ones we expect. This is because the IV fluid easily crosses your placenta during labour. If you notice this, don't be alarmed if baby loses more than 10 per cent of birth weight, as excess IV fluid distorts birth weight. Monitor his swallowing and poos closely to gauge how much he is getting instead.

What happens if you don't become engorged?

Some mums don't experience any engorgement even though their milk supply increases. This is better than becoming engorged as it tells you that baby is draining the breast well and your body knows how much to produce without going overboard. You'll know that he is getting enough by monitoring his nappies. (See page 70.)

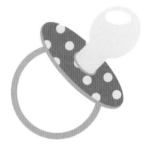

If you develop congestion after the first week, it is more likely due to some element of breastfeeding not working correctly, and if this is not addressed you can develop mastitis.

We'll look at how to avoid that in Chapter 18, so that you are fully prepared and know what to do if you need to act quickly. First, though, we'll cover latching challenges, as these contribute to sore nipples and poor breast drainage.

CHAPTER 17

HOW TO RESOLVE LATCHING CHALLENGES
WHAT TO DO WHEN IT'S NOT SIMPLE

This is an important chapter as there may be times when you try your best to get latching right but no matter how hard you try, you just can't seem to crack it.

It is important to remember that it is your baby who breastfeeds and is therefore responsible for a good latch. Provided you are holding and positioning him correctly, he should be able to latch without difficulty.

Variation in anatomy and birth stories often influence how well babies are able to latch; often these are quickly overcome, but sometimes intervention and breastfeeding tools are needed to enable him to feed well.

135

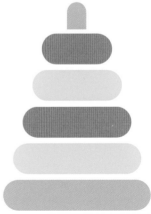

Common baby-related problems

➥ My baby won't open his mouth

• If you are holding his neck or jawline when latching, he won't open his mouth very wide. Ensure that you splay your fingers over his entire lower cheek. (See page 39.)

• Babies who fuss, arch and pull away from the breast usually have wind. If he is shaking his head left and right over the breast, pursing his lips or letting go just after latching, wind him before you try latching again.

➥ My baby keeps losing the breast

When your baby is born he may have a noticeable overbite from being curled up so tightly inside you. This makes grasping and holding your breast tricky.

• Create something firm for him to latch on to by shaping your breast (see page 54).

• If you are small-breasted you may not have enough breast for baby to hold on to, so try a nipple shield to start with as this is firm and easy for baby to latch on to (see page 180).

➥ My baby only latches on one side

As your baby turns and twists down the birth canal, tightness and tension can develop in his body, neck and head. This can mould and temporarily change the shape of your baby's head and make it uncomfortable to lie on one side.

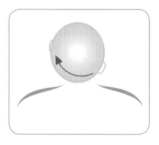 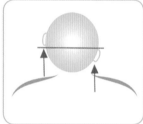

Looking at your baby from behind, you may notice that one ear is further back than the other, usually the one on the right side. This tightness makes lying on his right to feed from the left breast uncomfortable, which is why so many babies prefer feeding from the right side.

So, work with baby to find a position that feels good for him, such as the slide-over position as outlined on page 50. Or visit a cranial osteopath, who will work with baby to release residual tightness and tension from the birth (see page 185).

➙ Baby has a high-arched palate

Your breast and nipple need to get to the back of baby's mouth quickly when he latches so that he holds your breast in place. This is easily done if baby has a gentle dome-shaped palate (*Fig. 1*).

However, if he has a high-arched palate (*Fig. 2*) your nipple goes up first before moving back. The higher baby's arch, the harder it is for your nipple to get to the back of his mouth. Ideally he needs to scoop up more breast, but this will only be possible if he can open his mouth wide enough. As he gets bigger, this will become easier to do.

If he is little, you may find that your nipple becomes sore and looks like a D with the flat side close to his tongue and the rounded side close to his nose (*Fig. 3*).

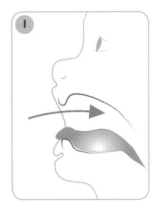
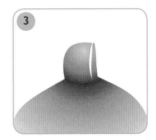
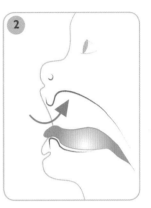

137

TIP

Use the Pinch and Pop latching technique on page 54, try feeding with nipple shields (page 180) and check for a tongue-tie, as it often goes hand in hand (page 138).

➤ Baby has a tongue-tie

A tongue-tie is an extra bit of vertical membrane that ties the base of the tongue to the floor of the mouth. It is quite common and is passed down through families. Not all tongue-ties cause significant problems but they can make breastfeeding more challenging.

(Fig. 1 and 2)
The degree of tightness and thickness varies, as well as where it ties. The tighter the tie and the closer to the tip of the tongue its placement, the more it affects baby's tongue movement necessary for draining the breast effectively without causing pain. To create room for your breast in baby's mouth, his tongue comes forward over his gum. If his tongue can't come out, your nipple won't go in very far and this is what causes common problems such as nipple pain and poor breast drainage. *(Fig. 3 and 4.)* The more pronounced the tongue-tie is, the more it will affect breastfeeding, speech and dental hygiene.

You'll know that your baby has a tongue-tie by:
• Looking at the shape of his tongue to see whether it is heart-shaped and can touch his palate. Also look for a string-like membrane under his tongue.
• Feeling the shape of his palate with your finger, your nail side on his tongue. His palate should be a gentle dome shape. If it is narrow, has a high arch or a little extra bit of height like a bubble, he probably has a tie.
• Feeling under his tongue with a clean, short-nailed index finger. Be very careful when doing this, as it will hurt if the tie is tight.

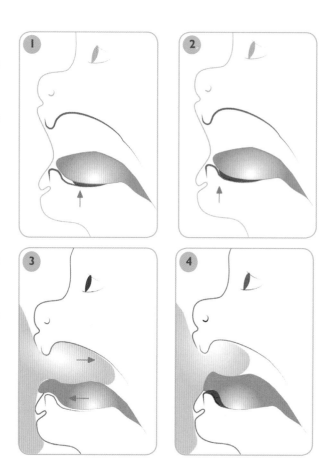

If you think your baby has a tongue-tie, find a doctor or dentist who specialises in ties and have it assessed. They'll assess it objectively and have the best skill set to divide it and minimise scar tissue developing, which creates more feeding problems. (See page 186.)

Common birth-related problems

Like us, your baby uses a lot of facial muscles when he eats, and these are all innervated by cranial nerves. His position in the womb, the length of your labour and any assistance he needs during birth can all irritate his facial nerves and make feeding tricky to start with.

Fast deliveries, which usually only take three hours from start to baby, involve strong contractions and a lot of force. This can cause tightness at the neck and base of head which often leads to baby chomping and feeding better from one side. Use the slide-over position (see page 50).

Slow deliveries often leave babies feeling quite tender. Be careful to support baby's entire head when latching, not just his lower jaw (see page 39). He may not do a wide gape to latch, so see my Brush and Clip technique on page 54 and use compression throughout.

C-section babies can either be very sleepy or very hungry. Sleepy babies will pose more latching challenges as they are full of mucus, so therefore they aren't hungry and don't open their mouth to latch. As your milk is delayed coming in due to the section, this is not good news and you need to get your baby interested in feeding or your delay will be greater. Try feeding with nipple shields (page 180) or hand-expressing to stimulate supply (see page 100).

Emergency C-sections have too many outcomes to get into but I want you to know that if breastfeeding is difficult after a long labour that ultimately resulted in an emergency section, it is not your fault. Some babies feed without any problem but others are tight and don't open their mouth properly, making you sore and feeding inefficiently. It will come right but don't be upset if baby needs a couple of bottle-feeds in the meantime.

Ventouse deliveries can leave your baby feeling more tight and sore on one side, so use the slide-over position (page 50). He may also be sleepier as jaundice is often prolonged and exacerbated by ventouse deliveries. Use the Brush and Clip technique to latch and monitor swallows to ensure things get better quickly.

Forceps deliveries lead to babies latching but not sucking. He might clamp down on your nipple but only feed for a few seconds because he can't mould your breast or keep it in place with his tongue. Most of my forcep babies start feeding using a nipple shield, as it is something firm for them to grasp on to. This allows baby to get your colostrum and milk directly from your breast until he can latch on his own (see page 180).

Common mum-related problems

When you latch your baby on to the breast, you are connecting physically, like two pieces of a puzzle. Sometimes the fit is not as good as it can be to start with, but this usually comes right over time.

→ **Small nipples (*Fig. 1*)**
Small nipples, less than 1cm diameter or the size of a pea, can experience a good deal of friction, especially if baby has a high-arched palate, is not scooping up enough areola when latching or loses the breast during the feed.

→ **Medium nipples (*Fig. 2*)**
Medium-sized nipples, usually 1.5cm or the size of a hazelnut, can become compressed and sore if baby is small 2.3kg (5lb), premature or has a small mouth in relation to the nipple.

→ **Large nipples (*Fig. 3*)**
Large nipples with a diameter of 2cm or more can be flat, pointy or inverted. The biggest challenge you have is getting the nipple and areola into baby's mouth. This is what I refer to as temporary incompatible anatomy.

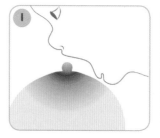
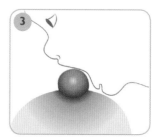
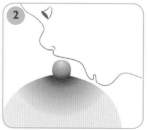

⇥ Inverted nipples (*Fig. 1*)

When filaments (little spring-like structures) in your nipple are very tight, your nipples are pulled into the breast. Sometimes with regular suction and feeding the filaments stretch and your nipple pops out. Other times, the filaments remain stubborn and your skin pulls away instead, leading to very sore nipples. You'll get a better idea of what your nipples will do by doing a simple pinch test.

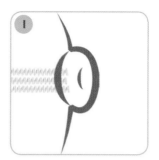

Some nipples look inverted but pop out when suction or pressure is applied just behind them. (*Fig. 2*)

True inverted nipples creep further back into the breast when you try to coax them out. Your baby may be able to latch if he scoops up enough areola but you may feel a sharp pulling pain. This is normal and a result of stubborn filaments. (*Fig. 3*)

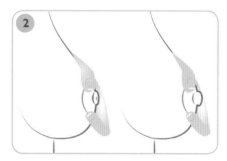

If it is bearable, continue feeding and over time it should feel more comfortable. If your nipples are bleeding, use a nipple shield or consider expressing and bottle-feeding for a while. Expressing allows you to control the level of suction applied to your nipple, so it will be more comfortable, but it also encourages filament stretching.

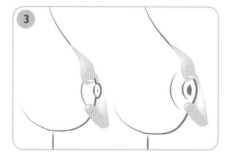

141

CHAPTER 18

HOW TO REDUCE SORE NIPPLES AND BREAST PAIN
FIND YOUR WAY TO PAIN-FREE FEEDS

There are often very clear, simple causes that lead to nipple damage and breast pain. Simply put, nipple damage is usually caused by poor positioning, latching or both, and breast pain is usually caused by poor breast drainage.

There is a lot of crossover between sore nipples and sore breasts, in that if your baby isn't positioned well, your nipples will get damaged and he won't drain the relating area of the breast. Sometimes nipples and breasts get sore independently of each other and I'll cover those issues at the end of this chapter.

As soon as your breasts become congested, hot, red or inflamed, you need to remember the following:

Apply ice to reduce swelling.

Take ibuprofen* to reduce systemic swelling.

Drain your breasts effectively.

speak to GP before taking ibuprofen

Why do nipples get sore?

Friction on the nipple caused by a poorly positioned baby, pump or nipple shield is the most common cause.

Quick illustration
Imagine that your thumbnail is your nipple. Put your lower lip on your thumb cuticle, pop your thumb into your mouth and have a suck. Can you feel your tongue brushes over your thumbnail (would-be nipple)? (*Fig. 1*)

Now put your lower lip on the first knuckle of your thumb, pop your thumb into your mouth and have a suck. Can you feel that your tongue hardly touches your thumbnail (would-be nipple)? (*Fig. 2*)

When you line baby up nose to nipple, baby gets enough areola for a good latch.

Why do breasts get sore?

You'll find that there are lots of different aches and pains that you experience just before a feed, during a feed and after a feed. Most of them are nothing to worry about and are just down to your breast getting used to its new role.

Shooting pains, tingling and angry ants are some of the ways mums describe a forceful let-down at the start of the feed. It usually coincides with over-production and is worse at the start of the feed, but this settles down during the feed and goes completely after a few weeks.

Your breasts ache, throb and swell when they aren't drained properly. If the skin on your nipple is cracked, you can also get a bacterial or thrush infection in the breast. All of this can be avoided by feeding according to your breast size (see page 30) and using the subtle troubleshooting position changes that we'll cover here.

143

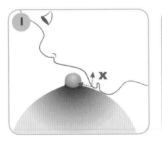

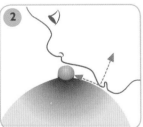

TIP

Sore nipples and breast pain are easily avoided by good positioning during the feed.

Upper nipple base wounds

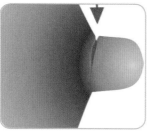

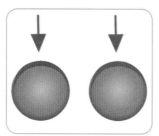

→ **Common causes**
• Your baby slips downwards during the feed: Baby's top cheek and the corner of his mouth move closer to the nipple, gradually wearing down the skin on the top half of your nipple. (*Fig. 1*)
• Your baby rolls away from the breast during the feed: The upper part of your nipple is repeatedly pulled away from the breast. Over time, this can tear or crack. (*Fig. 2*)

→ **Other causes**
• A poorly positioned pump funnel or nipple shield that rubs against the nipple.

144

TIP

It may be hard to see these hairline cracks but you will know that they are there if you have an intense initial burning when baby latches.

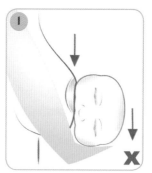

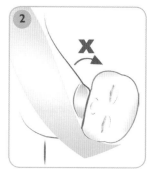

Mastitis in the upper half of the breast

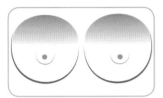

This is probably the most common area of congestion and mastitis development. It is so easy to avoid developing it when you ensure that both of baby's cheeks touch the breast evenly during the feed. This allows baby to drain the entire breast well.

↪ **Common causes**
• Your baby slips downwards during the feed: Baby can't drain the upper half of your breast properly. (*Fig. 1*)
• Your baby rolls away from the breast during the feed: The upper half of your breast pulls out of his mouth and affects drainage. (*Fig. 2*)

↪ **Other causes**
• A tight top that you lift to feed which cuts into your breast, restricts milk flow and drainage.

145

TIP

It is so easy to let baby slip downwards or pull away from the breast when you feel more relaxed about breastfeeding. These wounds and blockages are easy to resolve and avoid by keeping baby at the right height and close to you.

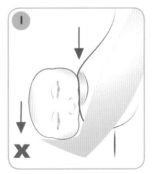
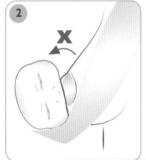

Lower nipple base wounds

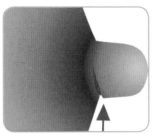

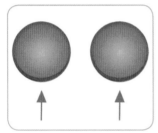

↪ **Common causes**

- Your baby moves up after latching: When your shoulders rise up they lift baby and get his lower cheek closer to the nipple. (*Fig. 1*)
- Your baby's lower cheek doesn't touch your breast (*Fig. 2*)
- Your post-birth baby bump gets in his way and prevents him rolling under your breast. (*Fig. 3*)

↪ **Other causes**

- A poorly positioned pump funnel or nipple shield that rubs against the nipple.

TIPS

Keep your shoulders relaxed.

•

Lift your breast with rolled-up muslin.

•

Check that baby's lower cheek touches your breast.

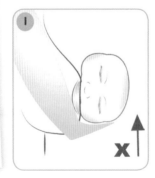

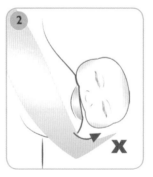

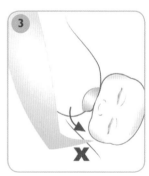

Mastitis in the lower half of the breast

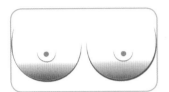

Mastitis in this part of the breast will come as a nasty surprise as it is so easily to miss, especially if you are large-breasted. As a rule of thumb, always position baby a smidge lower than you think he needs to be or use a small mirror to check that his lower cheek is in contact with your breast.

↪ Common causes
- Your breast moves downwards: this happens so easily if you lift the breast before lining up baby. When you let go of the breast, it moves downwards to its natural resting position and falls out of baby's mouth. (*Fig. 1*)
- Your baby's lower cheek rolls away from the breast when you swap arms. (*Fig. 2*)
- Your baby isn't positioned under your breast enough. (*Fig. 3*)

147

TIPS

Move baby and your breast down together after latching.

•

Roll baby under your breast more.
Feed in the underarm position.

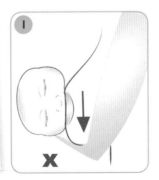

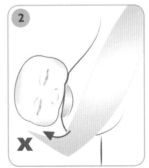

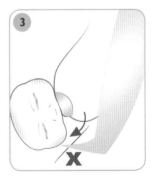

Inner nipple base wounds

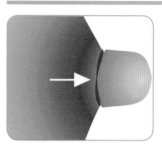

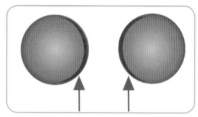

⇸ Common causes
• His lower lip is too close to your nipple when latching. (*Fig. 1*)
• His head is in the crook of your arm: When you swap arms, support baby's head with your wrist, so that his lower lip stays away from the nipple base. (*Fig. 2*)

⇸ Other causes
• Your baby has a tongue-tie.
• Nipple cream makes your areola slippery.
• Your baby is curled like a banana rather than his back being nice and straight.

TIPS

Line him up with his upper nose to your nipple.

•

Bring him straight on to the breast.

•

Bring his body into the breast – not his head.

•

Keep him in the same position when you swap hands.

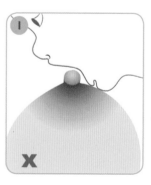
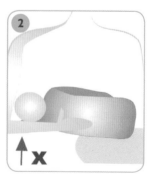

Mastitis the inner half of the breast

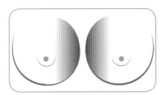

You need to pay attention to where your baby's lower lip is when latching and during the feed. If it creeps closer to the nipple during the feed or overshoots the areola, your baby won't be able to effectively drain the inner half of the breast.

↪ **Common causes**
• Your baby is positioned too close to the nipple when latching on to the breast. (*Fig. 1*)
• Your baby's head is in the crook of your arm, which pulls his lower lip closer to the base of your nipple as you relax into the feed. (*Fig. 2*)

↪ **Other causes**
• Your baby has a tongue-tie and, even with the best position and attachment technique, he struggles to drain the area of the breast close to his lower lip.

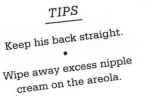

TIPS

Keep his back straight.

•

Wipe away excess nipple cream on the areola.

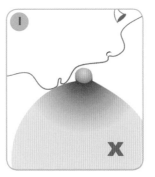

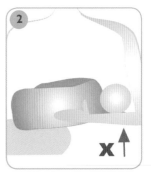

Outer nipple base wounds

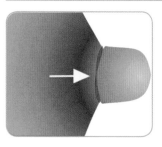

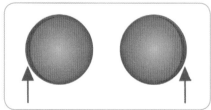

→ **Common causes**
- You line up the tip of baby's nose with your nipple. (*Fig. 1*)
- Your baby's legs are curled around your side. (*Fig. 2*)

→ **Other causes**
- You move your breast before getting baby into position.
- Your baby has a high-arched palate.

TIPS
Line up baby's upper lip to the nipple.

•

Keep his body in a straight line.

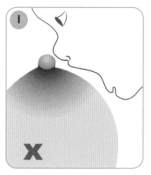

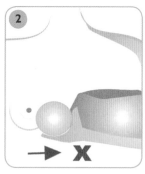

Mastitis in the outer half of the breast

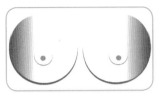

This part of the breast has excess breast tissue which extends into your armpit, called the Tail of Spence. When your breast is too full for baby to drain, this part of the breast is last to be drained and flares up.

↦ **Common causes**
• You line up the tip of baby's nose with your nipple and baby is too far from the nipple to latch well. (*Fig. 1*)
• Your baby's legs are curled around your side. (*Fig. 2*)

↦ **Other causes**
• You move your breast before getting baby into position.
• Your baby has a high-arched palate.

TIPS

Position him when your breast is at rest.

•

Compress your breast during the feed.

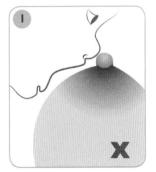

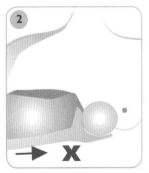

Nipple tip and entire base wounds

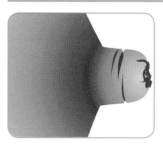

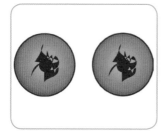

⇀ Common causes

• Wounds like this are caused when the nipple is forced into a space too small to accommodate it. The entire nipple comes into constant contact with the sides of whatever it is being put into. (*Fig. 1*)

⇀ Other causes

• Your nipple is large in relation to baby's mouth (see page 140).
• Your baby has a tongue-tie (see page 138).
• Your nipple shield is too small (page 180).
• Your pump funnel is too small (page 106).

TIPS

Express and bottle-feed until baby is bigger.
•
Check whether he has a tongue-tie.
•
Try bigger nipple shields.
•
Compress your breast.

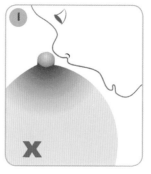

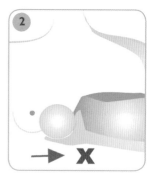

Extensive mastitis affecting the entire breast

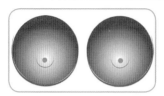

Entire breast inflammation is overwhelming, scary and incredibly sore. Your body is telling you that there is a problem with overall breast drainage rather than just one area that becomes congested with minor drainage inconsistencies.

↪ **Common causes**
• Oversupply issues as well as bacteria can cause this intense form of breast pain and congestion.
• Your entire breast fails to be drained properly as only your nipple is affected, rather than a wider circumference of your areola.

153

TIPS

Try a wider pump funnel.

•

Remove silicon insert if you have one.

•

Check that your nipple is centred to pump and shield.

•

Compress your breast.

Sore nipples without wounds

It's hard to know how much pain is 'normal' when you haven't breastfed before and there aren't any wounds to indicate what the problem is.

Breastfeeding shouldn't be sore. If it is, there is a problem that can be corrected. Please don't soldier on in pain. There is an easier and more enjoyable way to breastfeed your baby.

TIPS

Line up baby's upper lip to the nipple.

•

Keep his body in a straight line.

↪ **Blocked nipple pore**

When you have a blocked pore, you will notice a white milk dot or blister on your nipple tip. It may look yellow in colour if it has been there a while and may be more noticeable at the end of the feed.

What can I do?

• Apply a hot, wet facecloth to the nipple before you feed. This will soften the excess dead skin on the nipple and help the milk come through.
• Compress the breast to help push milk down and through the blocked pore.
• If you are clearly able to see where the blocked pore is, you can undermine the integrity of the skin by carefully scratching over it with a sterile needle. You shouldn't feel the needle on your nipple. If you do, you are applying too much pressure and can hurt yourself.
• Take lecithin to clear your milk ducts (see page 181).

↣ Vasospasm

When you have vasospasm the capillaries in your breast and nipple spasm and stop the blood flow temporarily. You can feel a tightening in the nipple and breast before experiencing a sharp pain. Often your nipple becomes white before turning very red. A throbbing sensation or feeling of angry ants inside your breast lasts for a few minutes before settling.

Vasospasm is often misdiagnosed as thrush. The difference is that vasospasm happens on an ad-hoc basis during the day or is triggered by a drop in temperature and is not the constant burning sensation that you get with thrush.

What can I do?

• Keep your breasts warm.
• Apply a hot water bottle to the nipple before and after the feed.
• Apply pressure with the palm of your hand when the nipples spasm.
• Reduce your caffeine intake.
• Increase your intake of calcium-, magnesium- and potassium-rich foods.
• Speak to your GP about taking a course of nifedipine.

↣ Thrush

Thrush nipples are very pink or raspberry red. The skin may be dry and itchy and the nipple and areola may have a shininess to it.

Your nipples will sting and burn throughout the feed without respite. Mums often describe this as the feeling of sandpaper, a cat's tongue or broken glass being massaged into the nipple during the feed. The pain is intense but the nipple is round at the end of the feed, which indicates a perfect latch.

After the feed the pain may escalate and having anything in contact with your nipples will send you into overdrive.

What can I do?

Speak to your GP or health visitor so that they can prescribe miconazole or clotrimazole cream.

Natural remedies include:
• Probiotics for you and baby.
• Citricidal soaks (see page 182).
• Colloidal silver spray from your homeopath (page 182).
• Cut sugar and alcohol out of your diet.

Sore breasts and mastitis

When your breasts aren't emptied properly or frequently enough, a backlog of milk develops and causes pain in your breast. If you don't deal with this, the pain escalates and you develop an infection and flu-like symptoms, which we call mastitis.

Your GP will give you antibiotics to help you feel better but, if possible, it is better to take steps to prevent mastitis, as it will make you really feel awful. The easiest way to do this is to get your baby positioned properly and feed according to your anatomy.

Apart from the positional problems that we have looked at, there are indirect causes that can lead to breast tenderness.

↝ **Missed feeds**

Your body likes rhythms and patterns; so the sooner you can establish a workable breastfeeding pattern and stick to it, the better.

↝ **Stretching baby between feeds too early**

If you are small-breasted or your baby is little and has a restricted stomach capacity, you will run into problems quickly as your breasts won't cope with having too much milk and your baby will only be able to take off a set amount at feeds.

Night nannies and maternity nurses boast about their ability to get babies to feed four-hourly within the first few weeks. This is a dangerous practice and I don't encourage it at all, especially for babies younger than four months – and even then it's questionable. Be sure to cover this point with them at your interview to be sure you get the right person.

156

TIP

Get the highest level of care with one of my girls at Miskin Maternity, see page 185.

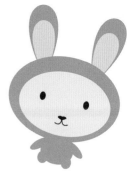

⇥ Baby sleeps through the night

Your body has an inbuilt safety mechanism in that when your milk supply is highest, which is typically between 1am and 4am, your baby is most wakeful. When your baby decides to sleep all night without warning, you'll wake to throbbing breasts rather than a hungry baby.

This is one time when I don't recommend waking a baby, as it is the beginning of a new chapter, however, you need to manage your supply so that you don't develop problems.

What should I do?

Here are three options to consider:

1. Wake baby to feed but push the feed closer to 7am by 15 minutes each day. What you are trying to do here is delay the feed a little each day, to encourage longer, healthy sleep habits, while managing your throbbing breasts.

2. If you find that your baby won't wake, you can express some milk off the breast. Express off just enough to feel comfortable. Reduce the amount you express by 10–20ml each day. If baby wakes early give him a little expressed milk to tide him over until his 7am feed.

3. Larger-breasted mums prefer to manage the breast pain and swelling by using ice packs until baby wakes and feeds. This doesn't work well for small cup sizes, though.

⇥ Ill-fitting clothing

Anything that pushes into the breast for long periods and creates a dent in the breast is going to impact breast comfort. Your nursing bra or even a breast shell that you wear to protect your nipples can cause blockages, too.

⇥ Sick babies

Breast-feeders are nose breathers. A stuffy or blocked nose can interrupt feeds as baby pulls on and off the breast to breathe. This can result in nipple pain but can also exhaust baby, and you may find that the breast is not well drained. Often sick babies have a suppressed appetite, which impacts drainage.

What can I do?

- Drop two to three drops of breast milk into baby's nose before each feed to decongest his sinuses.
- If baby is pulling at his ears, drop milk into them too.
- Feed your baby in an upright position, so that the mucus can drain from his sinuses during the feed.
- Raise baby's crib to lift his head for sleeps.
- Feed little and often as baby will manage short bursts and this will help manage supply.

CHAPTER 19

HOW TO MANAGE LOW MILK SUPPLY
HOW TO BOOST YOUR SUPPLY EASILY

There is so much 'noise' about breastfeeding online, in books and in conversations that it's hard to understand what is real or relevant anymore.

Simply put, your milk supply is governed by three key elements working well together – namely hormone function, glandular tissue and milk drainage. When there is a temporary misalignment/malfunction between these three key elements, your supply becomes suppressed until the problem is identified and resolved.

Permanent changes to one of these key elements, such as breast-reduction surgery, have a lasting effect on production and can lead to a true low milk supply.

More often than not, you will experience perceived or suppressed milk supply, which comes about when you don't feed according to your anatomy or if your perception of your supply is off-kilter.

The skinny on low milk supply

This is how to differentiate between perceived, suppressed and true low supply.

Perceived low milk supply refers to situations when you produce enough milk but don't have the confidence or tools to know that breastfeeding is going well.

Supressed milk supply refers to situations where your milk production is temporarily low due to poor milk transfer, unsuitable feeding patterns and bad advice.

True low milk supply refers to situations where medical conditions, breast surgery or lack of breast tissue permanently impacts the production of milk and results in low milk supply.

POOR MILK TRANSFER

In order to transfer and get your milk, your breast needs to fit snugly into baby's mouth so that his tongue, cheeks and palate in are full contact with your breast. When the fit between you and baby is not snug, baby has to work harder to get your milk.

He may run out of steam before emptying your breast, or hurt you, which often leads to a shortened feed.

Breastfeeding tools such as nipple shields can be used to fill the gap if baby has a high-arched palate, and compression can be used to increase milk flow. When you know what the problem is, the solution is easy to find too.

FOODS TO AVOID

Caffeine, aspartame, sage, peppermint and rosemary in large volumes

➼ Perceived low milk supply

When we think of a well-fed baby, images of a milk-drunk, floppy, relaxed baby who sleeps peacefully for hours on end, gains weight easily and never cries spring into mind.

This is certainly what we aim for but there are times when your baby gets what he needs but doesn't behave this way and shatters the illusion. You know that you have enough milk if your baby is gaining weight as he should be (see page 78).

Here are some possible causes of his unsettled behaviour:
• Growth spurts (page 82)
• Trapped wind (page 83)
• Poor milk transfer (page 159)
• Fast let-down (page 168)
• Tongue-tie (page 138)

➼ Suppressed milk supply

This is when you have enough functioning glandular tissue, healthy hormone production and/or breast drainage but you don't use one or all of them properly. It is a temporary glitch and can be rectified as soon as you find the key element that is out of sync.

How to recognise suppressed supply:
• Your baby struggles to regain his birth weight.
• He gains 100g or less each week and drops off his birth centile, looks skinny and doesn't grow out of his clothes as you would expect.
• He gains weight well in the first few weeks but then his weight gain trails off.

Assess these three elements below to find the missing link:

Glandular tissue

The less glandular tissue you have, the more frequently you need to feed, feeding from both sides so that you maximise glandular function. Feeding a hungry baby from a single breast when you are a small breast size is just not going to work.

Breast drainage

The more milk you drain from the breast, the more it will produce, so when trying to boost your supply, assess how well your baby feeds by monitoring how often he swallows. Your baby is usually able to drain the breast better than a pump if he feeds efficiently. When he doesn't feed efficiently, the pump often can and will do a better job.

If he does more than 10 sucks per swallow, milk transfer is poor. You are better off expressing to drain the breast and breastfeeding baby for comfort rather than nutrition until your supply increases and you resolve the root of the problem.

Hormones

A hormone imbalance can affect supply levels, so if you have any history of imbalances, get a blood test done to check that they are where they should be. If not, get your thyroid levels tested, as well as your vitamin D and iron levels. Ensure that you are eating a healthy well-balanced diet as well. (See page 25.)

Retained placenta can keep progesterone levels high, which will impact the efficiency of prolactin. So if your supply is slow to come in, double check that the placenta was intact and completely removed.

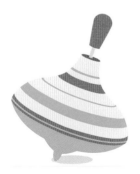

➜ True low milk supply

Unfortunately there are times when you may not be able to breastfeed exclusively but you may still be able to breastfeed in combination with formula.

Medical conditions such as diabetes, untreated low thyroid function, polycystic ovary syndrome (PCOS) and breast surgery can stifle milk supply. In these situations it is even more important for you to feed according to your anatomy or as though you were a small-breasted mum.

Which conditions might result in mums suffering a low milk supply?

• Severe polycystic ovary syndrome
• Low thyroid levels
• Diabetes
• Minimal breast tissue
• Breast-reduction surgery (cosmetic and medical)
• Losing a lot of blood after birth

I'm not going to go into detail here, because in these situations it is important for you to find local, one-to-one help so that you get the best care possible. I also want to stress that just because you have one or more of these conditions, breastfeeding may still work well for you, so give it a go.

Seek professional help to find the best way forward for you or your baby. If you like, you can try one of the mother's milk herbal teas that are on the market which support milk production, but they do tend to be very weak and don't always work as well as hoped.

Milk-boosting supplements

⇥ Fenugreek

This is a North African herb, typically used in curries and found in most health-food stores. It works to increase your prolactin levels, so that you have more milk available to drain. Your supply will only increase if you actively increase breast drainage simultaneously while taking it.

Fenugreek and fennel tea

Fennel is another good culinary ingredient that boosts milk supply and when fennel seeds are mixed with fenugreek, a potent combination is made. Only take this tea in emergencies. Here is a recipe for a tea you can make at home.

1 heaped teaspoon of fennel seeds
1 heaped teaspoon of fenugreek seeds
2 cups of water

Put all the ingredients into a saucepan and bring to the boil. Turn down the heat and simmer for 10 minutes. Pour through a strainer and discard the seeds, then drink.

⇥ Shatavari

This is another popular herb used to boost milk supply. Speak to your local herbalist before taking this because it is not as well known as fenugreek and you want to be sure that it is suitable for you.

> ### TIP
> Always check with your herbalist or GP before taking any supplements.

> ### *FOODS TO IMPROVE THE QUALITY OF YOUR MILK*
>
> If you just can't boost your supply, focus on altering the quality of your milk by introducing lots of foods high in good fats into your diet. Things like oily fish (salmon and mackerel), coconut products such as yogurt, nut butters (cashew, hazelnut), mixed seeds and ground seed pastes (tahini). As your milk become more calorific, your baby will gain more weight and feel more satisfied after feeds.

Six highly effective milk-boosting plans

 ### Switch nursing

When you have a let-down, milk is released in both breasts simultaneously. Rather than leaving your baby to suckle on an empty breast while your alveoli refill, offer him the other side so that he gets the milk waiting to be drained. This will increase the volume of milk drained at a feed and increase your supply naturally.

 ### Afternoon pick-me-up

This is great when your supply is low and you are cluster-feeding all afternoon and into the early evening.

Take one to two fenugreek capsules at lunchtime for three days, then stop taking them. This will lift your late-afternoon supply. You can increase the amount to three capsules if your supply does not pick up, but gauge how your body responds to one before doing so to avoid developing mastitis.

Feed baby well each time he asks for food by:
• feeding from both sides
• compressing
• waking baby to feed when he goes to sleep during the feed

The more you feed and drain from your breasts, the quicker your supply will increase.

 ### Three-day booster set

Take one fenugreek capsule three times a day. Increase to two or three capsules three times a day if you don't see an increase in your milk supply within 24 hours. Take fenugreek for three days and then stop for four to assess whether your supply has increased.

While taking fenugreek, ensure that baby drains the breast well. If you develop congestion, tenderness or a lump in the breast, stop taking the fenugreek until the problem is resolved.

If you just don't have the time or headspace to focus on boosting your supply during the week, do a two- to three-day intense booster set over the weekend when your partner is around (see plan 4, overleaf).

TIP

Short, effective boosts are much better than long-drawn-out processes, which aren't suitable or sustainable for busy mums.

4 Incredible three-day booster set

The intense three-day booster set is better to do over a weekend when your partner is home to share the load. Order in, plan a duvet day and movie weekend because you are going to be busy!

It includes:

- Three fenugreek capsules three times a day with meals
- Feeding from both sides at least every two to three hours
- Stealing the milk strategy (see plan 5)
  Or:
- Power-pumping sessions twice a day (plan 6) in addition to your feeding.

Your aim is to boost your supply from the inside using fenugreek capsules while physically draining all the milk you produce, as soon as it is produced, in order to produce more. It is the daddy of milk-boosting strategies and one that is sure to work.

5 Stealing the milk strategy

In order to produce more milk you need to drain more milk from the breast. Expressing after a feed is not always useful, though, because the pump is not as effective as baby at draining the breast. You are therefore less likely to drain any milk off the breast after a feed if baby typically 'empties' the breast well at feeds.

By expressing both breasts for 10 minutes each, while compressing throughout, you will be able to access and express the 'easy milk'. The resting time between the end of your express and baby's feed is enough for your breasts to refill. Just be sure to time your expressing so that you finish 20 minutes before baby's usual feed is due. If baby wakes sooner, just breastfeed as you normally would and top up baby with the expressed milk you accumulated.

WHEN BABY FEEDS

Feed him from both breasts.

•

Compress throughout the feed to ensure he doesn't have to work too hard.

•

Switch between breasts as necessary when baby no longer swallows.

When you find that baby is no longer swallowing and has fed from both breasts twice, offer him the milk you expressed before the feed.

•

Always check with your herbalist or GP before taking any supplements.

6 **Power-pumping sessions**

This is probably best done at the beginning of the day, before your baby's first feed and while your partner is home, and at the end of the day when baby is asleep.

To power pump you:

- Express both breasts for 10 minutes each while compressing.
- Then rest for 10 minutes.
- Pump for 10 minutes on each again.
- Repeat this cycle as many times as you can in an hour.

If you are using a single pump you will only get two cycles in an hour, and if you are double pumping and expressing both breasts simultaneously you will get three cycles in an hour.

How to wean baby off formula top ups

If you are using formula top ups it is probably because you are worried that baby is not getting enough milk from your breast. Hopefully you have rectified this by boosting your supply but if you or your partner are still worried, follow these steps.

1 Have your baby weighed weekly to ensure that he is gaining weight.

2 Once he consistently gains more than 30g a day, reduce the top-up by 10ml every other day.

3 As your supply increases, his weight gain will be consistent, even though you drop small amounts of top up.

165

TIP

Don't reduce formula top ups until your baby is gaining more than 30g each day.

CHAPTER 20

HOW TO MANAGE OVERSUPPLY
WHAT TO DO WHEN YOU HAVE TOO MUCH MILK

Supply issues directly influence so many areas of your day with baby that it is important to get them under control as quickly as possible. While an imbalance of hormones can contribute to over-production, more often poor advice and incompatible breastfeeding patterns are the cause.

If you have read the chapter on how to feed your baby in the first three months (Chapter 8), you will know that feeding according to your breast and baby size is important to create a balanced milk supply.

With infinite variations of mum-and-baby combinations, I know that not all mums or babies will experience the same issues, and on paper you may not even look like an oversupply candidate but your instinct tells you differently.

In this chapter, I want to help you identify the root of the problem and give you practical tools to bring your supply in line with baby's needs.

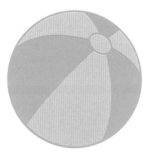

How to recognise when you have an oversupply

This is not an exclusive list and if you experience some of these points but both you and your baby are happy, there is no need to change anything.

➥ Your symptoms
- Your nipples are sore because baby insists on nipple-feeding.
- Your breasts are full, achy and sore all day.
- You are constantly on the verge of developing mastitis.
- You develop mastitis easily.
- Your breast pain keeps you awake at night.
- Your baby is older than three weeks and you still feel engorged throughout the day.

➥ Baby's symptoms
- Your baby gulps, coughs and splutters at the breast and hardly drains it.
- He struggles with wind and indigestion and grunts and moans all the time.
- His poos are spinach-green, slimy and explosive.
- He does 12 dirty nappies a day and cries in pain with each movement.
- He gains more than 7oz or 210g each week consistently.

When oversupply is normal

Your breast size and storage capacity can lead to oversupply symptoms.

➥ Small breasts
If you are producing enough milk to satisfy a hungry baby, what you are experiencing is very normal. Things will settle down once he feeds less frequently and needs less milk. This usually happens between three and four months, when your prolactin levels drop and baby grows at a slower pace.

➥ Medium- and large-breasted mums
As you have more storage capacity, you are likely to produce more milk than your baby needs. This will only be a problem and need addressing if you develop recurrent blockages or mastitis.

167

FOODS TO AVOID

Fennel, fenugreek, milk thistle, Shatavari

The difference between oversupply and forceful let-down

The key difference is that you can have a fast and forceful let-down without a lot of milk. You will know that you have a forceful let-down rather than an oversupply if your baby coughs and splutters at the breast at the start of the feed then drains both your breasts completely but is still not full.

You know that you have a fast or forceful let-down as a result of an oversupply when your baby coughs and splutters throughout the feed, doesn't drain your breast effectively but seems knocked out on your milk.

Both of these can lead to your baby being very windy and uncomfortable after feeds as he will swallow air in both instances.

Green poos are more likely when you have an oversupply but may also be a symptom of forceful let-down as your baby feels full (having swallowed a lot of air) before he really is and stops feeding.

Manage a fast and forceful let-down

Prevention is better than cure, so, where possible, take baby off your breast quickly when you feel a let-down coming. Direct the fast spray into a muslin cloth or apply pressure over your nipple and areola with your palm, pushing inward, to curb the let-down.

You can try feeding with nipple shields at the start of the feed, as this will moderate your flow and break the milk stream. If your supply is very high, you may find that this only makes a slight improvement.

Don't express regularly or before a feed, as this will only exacerbate your oversupply problem. Consider reducing your supply by block feeding (see opposite) and taking sage supplements.

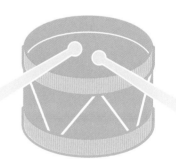

Three ways to lower your supply

1 Feed from both sides (good for small breasts)

By taking a bit off each breast at each feed, your body will only replace the small amount that baby removes but your breasts will feel more comfortable.

Switch-nurse, offering each side for five minutes before swapping over. Move back and forth between breasts until baby is full and both sides feel evenly drained. Your breasts may still feel full but this fullness helps your body regulate production (see page 21).

Your baby may get too much foremilk for a couple of days but this will soon pass. Use Colief drops with each feed to help him digest the excess lactose if his poos turn green and his tummy seems sore (see page 184).

2 Block feeding (good for medium and large breasts)

Feed baby as often as he needs but only offer one breast within the three-hour block. Apply ice packs to the side that you are not feeding from and express just enough to take the edge off the full side if you need to. Then offer only the other side for the following three hours and monitor the unfed side.

If your supply doesn't dip after 24 hours, you can increase the period of time you offer one side to four, five or six hours, until your supply slows down. Always reassess your supply after 24 hours and decide whether to continue with your block-feeding strategy or not.

3 Express to regulate supply

When your baby breastfeeds he has to swallow the milk that sprays into his mouth regardless of how hungry he is. In these instances, it is best to restrict drainage by expressing, as you will be able to control how much is drained at each feed.

Simply calculate how much baby needs at each feed (see page 111) and express a little more than he needs at regular times during the day. By controlling how much you drain, you can teach your body what to produce.

If you find that you need to express more than baby needs at each feed, do this so that you don't develop mastitis. Then, once you are in a rhythm, gradually reduce the amount that you express until you meet baby's needs.

4 Herbal remedies

If you are still struggling with oversupply, speak to your local herbalist about using sage, peppermint, rosemary, lemon balm and thyme to reduce your supply. Often they will be able to make up a tincture or tea using these ingredients.

CHAPTER 21

HOW TO INTRODUCE A BOTTLE WHEN YOUR BABY SAYS NO!
TIPS THAT REALLY WORK

When your baby is little he has an involuntary suck reflex and will happily suck on a bottle, but this reflex becomes voluntary by 12 weeks, sometimes earlier. This, along with changes to his usual routine or day, which make him insecure, can lead to bottle refusal.

There is a gentler way of introducing a bottle into your routine than running for the hills with a box of Kleenex and leaving a determined granny or dad to get the job done! Here's how I like to do it.

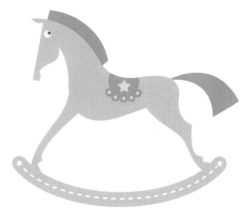

What to know before you start

The first thing to say is that every baby is different and it is important to tweak any tips in this chapter to suit your little one. Locking horns really isn't an option as this just stresses you both out and results in unnecessary tears.

Often babies will associate stress and anxiety with bottle-feeding after a period of unsuccessful introduction – or reintroduction. When you are under pressure and have a limited amount of time to succeed, both you and baby can find yourselves feeling physically and emotionally frazzled. This is something I want to avoid at all costs.

Use any bottle with an easy flow, so that he can get milk easily.

Only offer your baby a bottle when you are both relaxed. There is no point forcing the issue if you have just moved or your baby is ill, as he will be very protective of breastfeeding during unsettled periods. You want things to be as stable and calm as possible because your baby needs to feel secure enough to let go of your breast.

TIP

The more you have tried and failed with the bottle before, the more visible the bottle needs to be during the day.

171

Step 1: Introduce the bottle without confrontation

The more your baby sees the bottle during the day, the quicker he will accept that it is here to stay. You are developing a degree of familiarity in a calm and pleasant manner and when your baby recognises its worth, he will be less resistant to bottle-feeding. While you want it to be visible, it is important that it is not considered a toy, so only bring the bottle out of the cupboard at feeding times, unless you need to desensitise him first.

Have a prepared bottle on the table, sofa or close by at the beginning of each feed for a couple of days. Consider filling it with water and, when you are doing some winding, just give it a shake and show it to your baby – no feeding just yet.

If he has a meltdown at the sight of the bottle, do this for a few more days until he is not putting up a fight before you even offer it to him.

You may find offering your baby a bottle when he is surrounded by other bottle-feeding babies normalises bottle-feeding for your baby. It doesn't work instantly but can smooth over memories of confrontation he associates with bottles.

If you have had bad advice and forced the issue, maybe left baby with somebody else and the dreaded bottle, I would expect this reaction. What you are doing now is reintroducing it from a place of comfort and safety, such as your lap, and without confrontation.

You can have a bottle in the buggy when out for walks, in the cot and in pretty much any situation to desensitise him to the bottle. This reduces stress and encourages him to begin to see that the bottle really is just a bottle.

When your baby seems interested in looking, holding and playing with it, you are ready to move on to the next step.

> **TIP**
>
> The aim is not to feed him with the bottle, but to get him to tolerate the bottle.

Step 2: Encourage baby to accept the bottle without tears

Your baby may be fine with the bottle in the distance or as 'part of his day' but it may be very different when it becomes part of his feed. Start with a breastfeed to take the edge off his hunger, then offer the bottle and the breast again to reassure him.

Resistance is just part of the course and there is no point locking horns with him. When he sees that you are not forcing the issue, he will begin to trust you again. Calm him down with a feed and try again.

Ensure that he is relaxed and winded before offering the bottle. You can increase the number of feeds you practise at when your baby tolerates the bottle with little resistance.

At some point you may find that your baby is happy to chew on the bottle but doesn't suck it to get the milk inside. This creates a bit of stagnation so to move forward, you can try these things.

- You can give him a clean finger to suckle just before offering him the bottle. This should reinforce sucking and will encourage him to do the same on the bottle.
- You can offer him the bottle first before offering the breasts, especially if you can see that he is calm and happy but just not moving on to the next step.
- You can ask a familiar face to offer baby a bottle while you potter around. This can be your toddler, partner, mum, friend or similar. Your baby shouldn't feel threatened as you are still around, just occupying yourself with something else.

Step 3: Encourage small, regular feeds to start with

Now that your baby is happy to tolerate the bottle in his mouth without tears, you can encourage him to have small feeds. All you are hoping for is 10–20ml. Remove the bottle after a few sucks – it is better that you take the bottle away and leave your little one curious than try to keep the bottle in as long as possible.

Continued positive reinforcement is key and will keep your baby interested – even when he is pulling all sorts of faces. This is great practice for when you start introducing solids.

173

TIP

Don't give up if things don't move along quickly.

Step 4: Encourage baby to have a full feed

To encourage baby to have a bigger feed, breastfeed him before his bath and offer him a bigger bottle-feed afterwards in a darkened room, when he is more relaxed and sleepy. You may find that he takes the feed really easily but still wants to suckle from the breast before going to sleep. This is fine, and I would encourage you to go with it.

You can continue to offer a full feed after his bath or you can offer him a full feed at the 10pm feed (instead of breastfeeding) if things are going well. The choice is yours.

Once he happily takes the bottle from you without fuss, get your partner involved so that he can take over the late-night feed and you can get some extra sleep. Express in lieu of the feed.

↪ When it all goes wrong

If your baby gets to this stage and then seems disinterested, it's ok – he is probably just bored with it – but you can be confident that he can and will feed from a bottle.

Take a step back and allow Dad to do a bottle-feed while you are out of the house. You know that baby has been bottle-feeding, is comfortable with it and that you are not leaving him in the lurch to cry it out.

Alternatively, you can express a feed then go to a new environment and offer baby a full bottle-feed when out and about. By taking baby out of his comfort zone and into new surroundings, he is more likely to accept a different method of feeding once he has had some practice at home.

Sometimes the problem is that baby isn't hungry enough to be interested in feeding, so you could space out his feeds a bit and offer him a bottle-feed 30 minutes after his usual breastfeed is due (or before, if baby is hungry).

> ### TIP
> You have coaxed him and taught him what to do, so have the confidence to leave him to do what he needs to when you are not around.

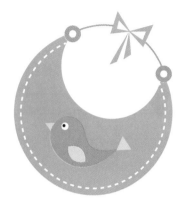

ESSENTIAL TIPS
TO GETTING BOTTLE-FEEDING RIGHT

Get your timing right; nobody likes to deal with confrontation or stubbornness when tired and desperate to get something else done.

•

Give yourself at least five weeks so that you are not under too much pressure.

•

If your baby refuses to drink breast milk from the bottle, try formula, cooled boiled water or a very weak, diluted juice.

•

Try offering him a bottle when he is very sleepy. Sit him upright so that the milk flow is slower and he is less likely to gag or throw up.

•

Remember, your baby is learning a new skill and it can be frustrating for the whole family.

•

Don't be hard on yourself or your baby; there is just no point.

As your baby grows and moves on to new things, your day will change quite a bit. It is tricky to know whether these changes are good, normal developmental changes or whether they are the start of a challenge. In the next chapter, I'll outline a few of the challenges that mums experience when breastfeeding an older baby.

175

CHAPTER 22

HOW TO MANAGE THE CHALLENGES OF FEEDING AN OLDER BABY
...WHAT NOBODY TELLS YOU

By three months you'd expect that breastfeeding is smooth sailing and problem-free, but some mums find that this is when all their problems start and breastfeeding comes crashing down, sometimes even to an abrupt, unexpected halt.

If you find yourself in this position, please be assured that you are not alone and that what you are experiencing is actually so common, it's quite normal.

The most common cause for everything turning on its head is that your baby has grown bigger and needs more breast to fill his mouth. However, as he is an old hand at breastfeeding, he is more interested in his surroundings and is not as focused as he once was.

As supply is driven by drainage, your supply starts to dip, making it a little trickier for him, and so the slippery slope begins.

The good news is that it is so easy to turn around and I'll show you how in this chapter.

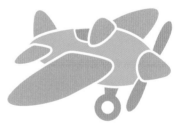

→ 12-week milk drop

At around 12 weeks your milk supply slows down to keep in line with your baby's slower rate of growth. This drop in supply ensures that you don't produce much more than your baby needs or develop blockages in the breast.

You may not notice that your supply has dropped to start with, but gradually you will find that he becomes fussier to the point of breast refusal. This is not breast refusal but a protest to sort out your supply, which is easily done (see page 158), and make it easier for him to get as much milk for as little effort as possible (see page 21).

If your supply is low and you have introduced formula without realising you were just experiencing a natural dip, try to wean yourself off formula top ups by boosting your supply (see page 163).

→ Baby loses the breast easily

It's difficult to differentiate this from baby's incredible social excitement to start with, but if you find that over time your baby's suck becomes weaker and he struggles to hold on to your breast, it is more than just being 'socially aware'.

Your baby may have an undiagnosed posterior tongue-tie that wasn't a problem before when he was small and his oral cavity provided a snug fit. Now that he has grown and his oral cavity has got bigger, it's harder to hold on to your breast when his tongue movement is restricted and the distance between his tongue and palate have increased.

You can improvise and use a nipple shield for a few weeks to bridge the gap between his palate and tongue. It's not advisable to have a tongue-tie divided after 12 weeks as it can lead to scar tissue developing and even more problems than before.

→ Baby drops off his growth curve

This is very upsetting, especially when you think everything is going well. It's difficult to say whether your supply is low or not, but I would suggest that you boost it anyway. Also, go back to basics and monitor how often baby is swallowing (see page 28). He may be working hard for his milk and burning calories rather than banking them.

TIP

If your baby is not draining your breast well, express to boost your supply or try using nipple shields to give baby a better grasp of your breast.

↪ Baby is too heavy to hold

As your baby gets bigger, your feeding position will need to change too. Often by three months your baby is able to feed with his bottom positioned on your outer thigh. However, you may still need to raise his bottom if he drags on your nipple and causes nipple damage. Keep his bottom close to you, so that he can drain your breast properly.

↪ Mastitis

As babies get bigger and you feel more confident about breastfeeding, your feeding positioning can often become sloppy. When one of baby's cheeks pulls away from your breast, you are more prone to developing blocked ducts and mastitis (see page 142) in that area of the breast. You may also be producing more milk than your baby needs; if so, see page 166 for advice on how to reduce your supply.

↪ Teething

You won't necessarily see any little teeth coming through to start with, but when they are on the move it can irritate baby and make feeds trickier. When teething, his gums will look red and inflamed. He'll be happy to gum away on your finger when you roll it over his gums, which may be hot to the touch and feel puffy.

Teetha, a homeopathic teething aid, is safe for young babies and is something to consider at this stage. You can offer baby something cold to chew on, but you will need to hold the teething ring for him, until his hand-to-mouth coordination allows him to do it himself.

↪ Distraction

As he gets older, baby will become more easily distracted during feeds. To keep him interested you can create distractions that he can only enjoy during a feed. A chunky necklace for him to play with during the feed or sitting a bright stuffed toy or material book on the sofa for him to look at over your shoulder are two quick wins. Sitting in a quiet room or corner when out and about makes feeds easier. You could also just do a quick feed in the car with some white noise or relaxing music before you get on with your shopping.

↪ Frequent night waking

While night waking and feeds are not ideal, it's normal for him to wake at night. If you find that it is becoming a habit or turning into a game, get him out of his crib, feed him well while sitting up and then put him back to bed.

You could also do a couple of split feeds during the day. Offer him some milk when he wakes, let him play and then offer some more milk when he looks tired or just before you put him down for a sleep. The more calories he gets during the day, the better he will sleep at night.

⇸ Snacking

Split feeds often carry negative connotations such as snacking, but it is an easy way to get milk into your baby so that he sleeps well at night. It won't interfere with daytime routines or naps when you don't count the second feed. Split feeding is a transition tool you can use until your baby is older and more able to cope with stimulation and longer wake times.

You are not regressing, failing or spoiling your baby, you are doing what works for an easier life, sleep and a more enjoyable experience.

⇸ Short feeds

He may only feed for five minutes before pulling off and looking disinterested. This is fine provided that he is not waking often and feeding all night. If he is, continue split feeding to ensure he gets enough milk to carry him through the day and night without becoming cranky.

⇸ Solids

Your baby is reliant on milk for the first 12 months of his life, because he is better able to absorb all the nutrients he needs and digest them easily. When you introduce solids too early, it can displace his milk intake and lead to a calorie or nutrient deficiency. See how to introduce solids on page 120.

⇸ Biting

Breastfeeding a baby with teeth doesn't sound like fun but it really won't change much unless he needs to bite to relieve irritation. Your baby's tongue covers his lower gum when feeding so, in theory, there is no reason for his teeth ever to come into contact with your breast.

With inflamed, sore and itchy gums, your baby wants to bite down on absolutely anything. Breastfeeding gives him a lot of comfort and, as the breast is already in his mouth, he'll unwittingly bite down to relieve discomfort. Your unexpected yelp may seem funny, turning it in a game. He doesn't understand that he has hurt you and is keen to try it again, to see if he gets the same reaction.

To reduce the chance of biting, apply some Calgel or Bonjela to his gums five minutes before a feed. Offer him something cold to chew on like a frozen teething ring or a block of frozen breast milk in a net dummy that is used for solids. When feeding, take him off when he becomes fussy or you can feel him pull his tongue back to expose his gums and little tusks.

Older babies often bite more frequently if your supply is low and they are bored. Offering the breast repeatedly when baby refuses will also lead to him latching and biting in protest, even if his feed only lasted three minutes.

USEFUL PRODUCTS
HOW AND WHEN TO USE THEM

Feeding tools

Nipple shields look like little silicon sombreros (Mexican hats) with a bit cut out on the side where baby's nose goes. They fit over the nipple and create a firm teat for baby to latch on to and suckle. Latching is simple as baby is lined up mouth to shield and comes straight on to the breast.

Nipple shields come in three sizes if you use the Medela brand. It is important to get a size that suits first your nipple then baby's mouth. However, you may find that the size that works for you is too big for your baby. In which case you probably need to express until he can latch or is bigger to avoid nipple damage caused by small shields.

Get a small nipple shield if your nipple is the same circumference as your little finger. Get a medium nipple shield if your nipple is the same circumference as your middle finger, and get a large one if it is the same circumference as your thumb. Once your baby has latched on to the breast, monitor his suck-to-swallow ratio, to ensure that he is getting milk easily.

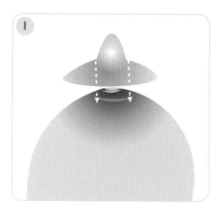

When to use:

You	Baby
Inverted nipples	Twins
Flat nipples	Forceps delivery
Sore nipples	Baby who was back to back

> **TIP**
>
> Nipple shields allow your baby to get milk directly from your breast. They are great tools and cut out the need for expressing, bottles and formula.

Useful products for common breastfeeding problems

→ **Mastitis (and engorgement)**

Ice packs

Apply ice packs to your breasts as soon as they become inflamed or red in colour. This will reduce swelling and create room for your milk ducts to open and allow milk flow and drainage. Anything from the freezer that will cool your breast will work. There is no need to buy anything special; a bag of frozen peas works a dream if you are caught off guard.

Hot water bottle or wheat bag

Apply heat to your breast just before a feed to encourage blood flow to the infected area and encourage milk flow for better breast drainage. Use in combination with cold packs to prevent escalation of breast swelling and pain.

Ibuprofen

It is a fantastic systemic anti-inflammatory and is safe to take while breastfeeding. If you feel that your engorgement is escalating, take 400mg of ibuprofen three times a day with meals to calm your breasts down. Check with your GP before taking it, especially if you are taking other medication or haven't had ibuprofen before.

Lecithin capsules

This is a soya-bean extract and a natural fat emulsifier that typically comes in 1200mg capsules. You can take one to four capsules a day to reduce blockages in the breast, if you suffer oversupply and recurrent episodes of mastitis, or have breast implants. While it is natural and usually perfectly safe, I suggest you have a word with your GP before taking it if you have any family history of allergies.

181

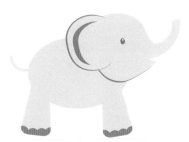

⇢ Sore nipples

Breast shells and manuka honey combination

Manuka honey is incredible stuff and, as it is a natural option, it is a favourite of mine. The higher the level of activity, the better it works. After feeding, rinse your nipples and apply Manuka honey generously to the nipple. To prevent the nipple sticking to your breast pad, wear a breast shell inside your bra. Wash your nipple well before feeding as honey can give your baby severe diarrhoea, which is dangerous for babies younger than 12 months.

Citricidal soaks

Citricidal is a grapefruit seed extract with powerful antibiotic, anti-fungal and anti-bacterial properties, which make it a great thrush remedy for breastfeeding mums. You can get a Citricidal solution from your health-food store and dilute 10 drops with 30ml of water to create a soak. Pour this mixture into an egg cup or similar, immerse your nipple and let it soak for a minute or so. Rinse well as it is extremely bitter and your baby will protest.

Cellular silver spray

This is another great natural remedy for thrush. Speak to your local homeopath, who will tell you how often to use it based on the severity of your symptoms.

Hydrogel discs

These are flat jelly-like discs that you wear against your skin, inside your bra and in combination with your breast pad. They cool and hydrate sore tender nipples and prevent unnecessary friction between your nipple and bra. They aren't absorbent so you still need to wear a breast pad to prevent leakage. For maximum effectiveness, keep them in the fridge.

TIP

You can find all of these products at www.geraldinemiskin.com

Hot, wet facecloth or flannel

To reduce bleeding, apply a hot, wet facecloth to the nipple prior to a feed to soften any dry skin or scabs, so that your baby doesn't pull these off during the feed and cause bleeding. Soothing and practical.

Lanolin

Lanolin promotes cell regeneration and is great for moist wound healing. Only use a quarter of a small fingernail between both nipples and wipe your areola well before latching baby. When it is overused it lubricates the areola and causes baby's lower lip to slip up to the base of the nipple. Stop using once your nipples have healed to prevent blocked pores, ducts and mastitis.

Multi-mam relief compresses

This is a lanolin-free option which is derived from plants. These compresses really soothe and rehydrate sore nipples, especially if they are kept in the fridge. Wear them inside your bra and breast pad between feeds until they dry out – usually 24 hours – then replace as necessary. Each box contains 12, so there are enough for both breasts for six days. Use in combination with salt-water soaks.

Nipple shields

Some mums use nipple shields to protect sore nipples and this is ok but it is not solving your problem, just covering it up. If you decide to use nipple shields to heal nipples, get some help to get baby off the shields and back on to the breast in a couple of days' time.

Salt-water solution

This might not sound great but it really works wonders. Add a couple of pinches of salt to a small glass of comfortably warm water. Pop your nipple into the glass to test how strong the solution is. You want your nipple to tingle, not burn. Add salt until you have the desired effect. Soak your nipple in the mixture for a minute or two after feeds, then rinse off the excess salt. Use in combination with Multi-mam compresses or hydrogel discs.

183

> *TIP*
>
> The trick here is to reduce inflammation quickly, so that you can drain your breast really well and stop mastitis developing.

⇢ Winding aids

Infacol

This can be used from day one to help baby bring up stubborn burps. Give him one squirt in his mouth before each feed – half a squirt into each cheek so that he doesn't spit it out. Use for at least 10 days in combination with good winding techniques before deciding whether or not to continue. Readily available in supermarkets and pharmacies.

Bubble-B-Gone (natural version)

It helps baby get rid of trapped wind naturally. Available online.

Infant probiotics

These support your baby's developing digestive system and are especially good after a C-section delivery, a course of antibiotics or if you think your baby has colic. Readily available in health-food stores.

Colief drops

They are synthesised lactase enzymes that help baby to break down the lactose in your milk. He shouldn't need these ordinarily but if you find that he struggles with a lot of gut pain or has green, explosive stools, it is worth trying with every feed for 10 days. Keep in the fridge once opened.

TIP

Always speak to your GP before giving your baby supplements.

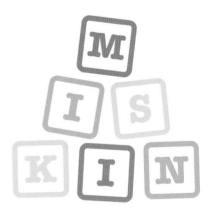

USEFUL SERVICES

⇢ UK services

Geraldine Miskin Consultancy

There's something special about having one-to-one help and I know that it makes a significant difference to breastfeeding outcomes. If you would like to book a consultation with me or one of my team, get in touch via my website. You'll also find breastfeeding products, videos and tips at www.geraldinemiskin.com

Miskin Maternity

If you want to breastfeed and are thinking about getting a maternity nurse, Miskin Maternity is the only place to go. We have hand-picked the very best girls and trained them up using the Miskin Method so that you get consistent advice based on your individuality. See www.miskinmaternity.com

The Bump Class

This is the best antenatal class available to mums who want unbiased, objective and practical information. The classes are run by experts in their fields, so you know that they are teaching you from experiences they encounter every day. See www.thebumpclass.com

Cranial osteopaths

This gentle form of therapy releases residual tightness in your baby's body, which helps him feel more comfortable. Having used it for years, I can highly recommend it as a gentle, non-invasive, baby-friendly treatment. Find your nearest practitioner online or by word of mouth.

Dr Ian Hay

A great supporter of breastfeeding and a consultant paediatrician at the Portland Hospital. See www.theportlandhospital.com

Dr Donald Gibb

London's leading private obstetrician provides the highest level of care for mums and mums-to-be. For an appointment see www.thebirthcompany.co.uk

Dr Joanna Helcke

A great source of inspiration and a powerhouse in the postnatal fitness industry. If you need inspiration or just some great tips to get active and learn how and when to exercise, she is the person to speak to. See www.joannahelcke.com

Dr Malcolm Levinkind

An amazing paediatric dentist who divides tongue-ties and upper-lip ties with laser. He is very knowledgeable and provides the highest level of care. For more information on how to reach him, see www.drlevinkind.com

Patti Good

The leading expert in emotional wellbeing for motherhood. Provides a number of services to ensure emotional preparation, health and wellbeing. See www.pattigood.com

185

⇢ International services

Baby-led weaning, www.babyledweaning.com
Invaluable advice and recipe books to ease your baby's transition to solids.

The Breastfeeding Network
This organisation provides clear and concise information about medications in their fact sheets section, making it easy to see whether they are safe to use while breastfeeding.
See www.breastfeedingnetwork.org.

Contented Calf Cookbook: Nourishing Recipes for Breastfeeding Mums, by Elena Cimelli
Eat your way to a great milk supply with this little gem of a book.

Dr Jack Newman
A great collection of breastfeeding videos to help you differentiate between sucks and swallows.
See www.breastfeedinginc.ca (see video section)

The International Affiliation of Tongue-tie Professionals
This organisation is committed to providing the most reliable and up-to-date information about tongue-ties and a list of where to go if you need your baby's tongue-tie assessed.
See www.tonguetieprofessionals.com.

KellyMom
This website provides objective, evidence-based breastfeeding information. A great resource for breastfeeding mums. See www.kellymom.com

INDEX

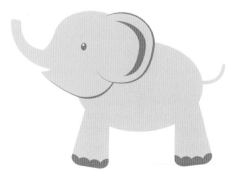

Acknowledgements

Writing a book that would make breastfeeding accessible to all mums has been a lifetime ambition of mine and it would not have come about without the help of an incredible group of people.

Firstly I'd like to thank all my wonderful clients who have been my greatest teachers. It has been a privilege to work with you.

I'd like to thank, Marina Fogle, Dr Ian Hay, Dr Donald Gibb and Deborah Turness for your encouragement, friendship and confidence in me. I hope this book does you proud.

A special thank you to my late father, a wonderful GP, for teaching me to always ask why and to find the root of the problem, rather than apply band-aid or one-size-fits-all therapy.

Thank you collectively to all my family and friends for enduring endless conversations about the book and for reviewing and critiquing my offerings. Patti, Marie, Tina, Marianne (Hart), Jana, Aretha, Lizzie, Monika, Freda, Christine, Margaret, Tiff and Cetti - you got the brunt of it so deserve a special mention!

To the Random House team, Samantha Jackson, Sophie Yamamoto, Helena Caldon, Catherine Knight and David Eldridge, you are all brilliant. Thank you for bringing this book to life.

Andy (Teakle), you have been an absolute lifesaver. Thank you for being the calmest, most capable designer I've had the good fortune to meet and at such a crucial time too.

To my husband and best friend, Neil. Thank you for being my greatest champion and cheerleader. Your love, patience and support have been invaluable to me and this book would not have come about without your help. Thank you. Thank you to my Lord and Saviour, Jesus Christ.